Potions & Notions

traditional remedies from far and wide

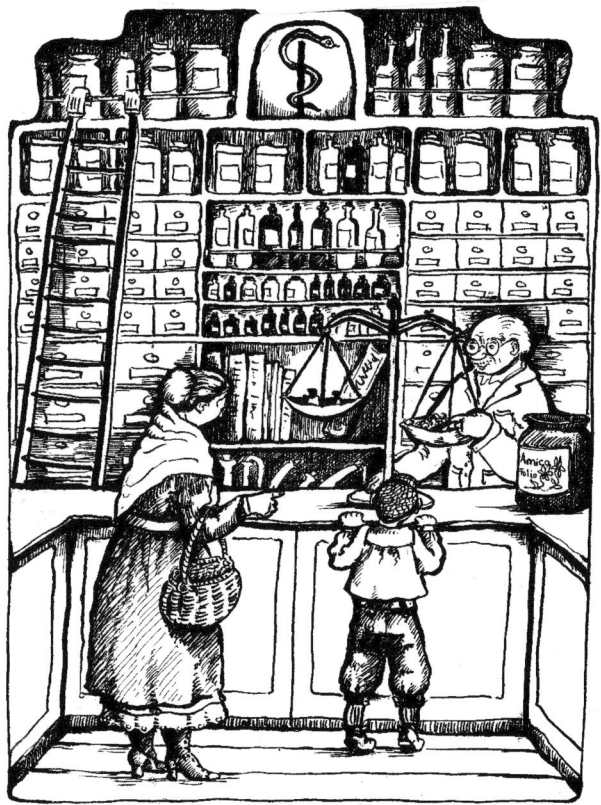

Christiane Franke

Published by Corridor Press,
The Arts Centre, 21 South Street,
Reading, Berkshire RG1 4QU,
England.

Tel: (0118) 901 5177
Fax: (0118) 901 5175
E-mail: corridor@dircon.co.uk

Printed and bound in Great Britain by Antony Rowe Ltd,
Bumper's Farm, Chippenham, Wiltshire, England

ISBN 1 897715 40 4

Corridor Press publications:
See It! Want It! Have It! (1992)
Bricks & Mortals (1994, reprinted 1994, 1996)
Moments of Glory (1996)
A Book of Cuttings (1997)
A Haystack of Young Poets (1998)

Under the imprint Corridor Poets (1997)
The Dark Larder Lesley Saunders
Einstein's Eyes Tim Masters
Scratched Initials Susan Utting
Small Infidelities Kristina Close

Potions & Notions

traditional remedies from far and wide

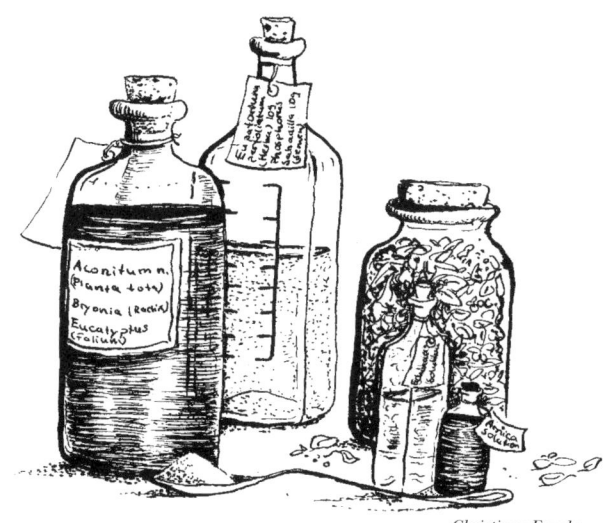

Christiane Franke

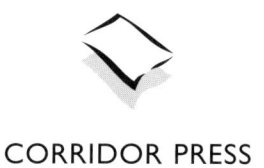

CORRIDOR PRESS

Acknowledgements

Our grateful thanks go as always to our loyal funders, Southern Arts and Reading Borough Council; to The Paul Hamlyn Foundation which gives invaluable support for training; the Reading Evening Post which sponsors our projects and gives us wide publicity; and Slough Borough Council for giving us financial support. We thank all our loyal volunteers for their continuing help and encouragement.

Thanks to Linda Barlow for local remedies culled from historic documents from the Berkshire Record Office; John Holden and Dermot O'Rourke for hours of research; Reading Girls' School for organising herbal workshops; Mrs Indira Desai for passing on 'grandmother's remedies'; Ursula Lyons, from Sudbury, Mass, for North American remedies; Michael Taylor for New Zealand remedies; and Jack Callow for Zimbabwean remedies.

The advertisements quoted in the chapter heads are from: *Secret Remedies: what they cost and what they contain* based on analyses made for the British Medical Association (1909) and *More Secret Remedies* (1912). Thanks to Dermot O'Rourke.

Thanks to:
Kathy Speers, of Woodley, for the recipe book of her Aunt Emily (Mrs Emily Taylor who died in the 1950s).
Gladys Bradford, of Newbury, for her father's book, *The Ship Captain's Medical Guide,* issued by the Board of Trade (1912).
Mrs Doris Hall, of Kingsclere, for loaning us *The R. E. P. Book, First Aid in Accidents and Ailments,* published by Elliman, Sons & Co, Slough, England (1903).
Margaret Skinner for lending us *Get Back to Nature and Live* by C W Aloysius Browne (c 1930).
Extracts also taken from *The Best Way: a book of household hints and recipes* (1907).

Thanks to:
Ronnie Rutherford for providing illustrations.
Wellcome Institute Library, London.
G R Lane Health Products Ltd, Gloucester, for advertisements from their archives.

Corridor Press is a member of the Federation of Worker Writers and Community Publishers

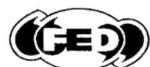 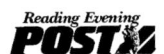

Contents

Foreword

Down the centuries, people have sought the means of healing and curing through natural remedies, the plants and herbs which grew around them, and the everyday materials which came to hand. In *Potions & Notions* we have collected some of those remedies, many of which are still in active use today.

People have passed on family wisdom, asked friends and relations, and dug out old books which have been in families for years. You will notice recurring patterns in traditional health care, whether it be from shaman or wise woman, herbalist or grandmother.

Like all the books we produce at Corridor Press, this is a truly community effort. Within Berkshire we have sought the stories of people from the many different cultures who have made their home here, and from their friends and families living abroad. This richly varied network of people is a microcosm of many communities.

Contributions have come from Australia to Zimbabwe, from pensioners to pupils. Our cover illustration was by Yasman Moghaddam, a schoolgirl from Iran, and several other illustrations are by Christiane Franke, from Germany. We would like to thank them and everyone who has contributed and hope you enjoy the wisdom, common sense and humour of these traditional remedies

Good health.

Alison Haymonds
Corridor Press

❐ Corridor Press is a non-profit-making community publisher funded by Southern Arts and Reading Borough Council and run by volunteers. We always welcome more people to join our book projects and take part in our training courses and workshops. You can contact Alison Haymonds or Linda Maestranzi at Corridor Press, The Arts Centre, 21 South Street, Reading RG1 4QU, Berkshire, or telephone (0118) 901 5177.

Contributors

Project group:
Liz Alvis
Tony Barham
Linda Barlow
Daphne Barnes-Phillips
Rosie Bass
Rose Cam
William Campbell,
Anne-Marie Dodson
David Downs
Mike Facherty
Alison Haymonds
Alexandra Henson
John Holden
Linda Maestranzi
Betty O'Rourke
Dermot O'Rourke
Beryl Pearson
Bill Tate
Annabel Wickens
Contributors
Ahood Al-Rehani
William Avery
Akhtar Aziz
Tony Barham
Linda Barlow
Daphne Barnes-Phillips
Lani Barwick
Trini Bello
Gladys Bradford
Jack Callow
Rose Cam
William Campbell
Dalip Chand
Audrey Cook
Anne-Marie Dodson
Doris from Woodley
Mike Facherty
Marjorie Pemble
Geraldine Friend
Gyosei College: Eiko, Sachiko.
Yoko and Yoshie
Joan Head
John Holden
Marguerite Hudson
Indian Yoga Group: Swami

Ambikananda, Kamala Tailor,
Tarala Jagirdar, Indira Desai,
Panna Desai, Vijayalaxmi (Viji)
Silvia Kufner
Linda Maestranzi
Teresa Mortl
Roisin O'Callaghan
Betty O'Rourke
Dermot O'Rourke
George Pottinger
Reading Girls School:
Rosie Bass, Frances Gregory,
Mary Parry and pupils
Carol Shepherd
Cyril Shuffle
Margaret Skinner
Mollie Smith
Isabel Sottomajor
Michael Taylor
Emma Thomas
Moy Trchalik
Agatha Walker
Carol Whelan
Annabel Wickens
Ala Zolkiewka
Cover
Designed by Damian Clarke
Yasman Moghaddam
Illustrations
Christiane Franke
Ruth Ezard
Joanne Lewington
Sabrina Mothin
Picture research
John Holden
Dermot O'Rourke
Transcription
Beryl Pearson
Proof reading and editing
Linda Barlow
William Campbell
Michael Facherty
Betty O'Rourke
Dermot O'Rourke
Editor
Alison Haymonds

In memory of Sue McGarry
(1963-1998)

Introduction

I welcome this latest community book with great enthusiasm and personal delight.

It is a very enjoyable, informative and amusing book which I hope readers will appreciate for years to come. Not only does it bring together contributions from all cultures and ages but it shows a variety of multicultural research combined with local knowledge, together making a really good, worthwhile publication.

I wish all contributors and Corridor Press success and hope the book is well received like so many of the other splendid publications.

Councillor Maureen Lockey
Reading Arts Forum

Head Start

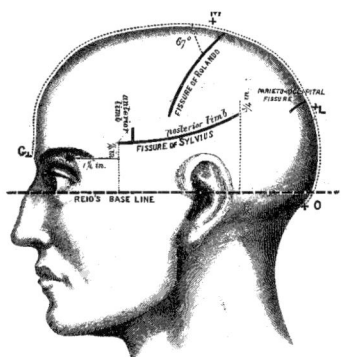

'The certain, trusty, genuine, right, honest Hair-Grower. There is no other. – Without "Tatcho" loss of hair is inevitable, but Mr Geo. R Sims has altered all that.'

Advertisement c 1912

Hair pieces

Sweet-smelling remedy

When I was a girl in Ireland, for some inexplicable reason my hair fell out in great patches, a condition called alopecia. I visited my doctor, a grumpy, bald-headed individual.

"How old are you?" he barked.

"Fifteen next week," I replied.

"I didn't ask you how old you would be next week," was his curt reply.

There was no word of comfort for the very sensitive nature of my predicament. However he did refer me to a specialist at a general hospital some miles away. There, to add to my embarrassment, I was prescribed ointment which smelt like rotten fish. I refused to go out.

Rosemary

My mother decided to go to a local herbalist. From him she bought a sweet-smelling ointment, whose main constituent was rosemary, which I used until, some months later, my hair had regrown. This was a more socially acceptable answer to my problem.

Roisin O'Callaghan

....

To prevent falling hair: Make an infusion of one and three-quarter ounces of nettle leaves (use the small annual nettle with tiny green-white flowers) in one and three-quarter pints of vinegar – put the nettle leaves in warm vinegar and let it stand for half an hour. Apply to hair.

....

Fern fronds and chalk

South African women would use fern fronds to help their thinning hair. These ferns grow like trees and the tops are like a palm tree with brownish fronds.

Women would burn them, mix them with chicken fat and apply the mixture to their hair like a balm. This was supposed to thicken the hair which made it easier to plait.

Women would also dig up chalk, mix it with water and literally cake the hair with it. It was almost like Plaster of Paris, reduced to powder when it was dry, and it just dropped off when it was rubbed. It nourished the hair and gave it a lovely texture. We also used castor oil on our hair for dryness.

Another method was to soak an onion in gin for about a fortnight and then use it as an astringent. This was also meant to stop baldness in men.

Rose Cam

A Cure for Baldness

I came to Reading in February 1945 and was appointed manager for John Millar at 2 Prospect Street, Caversham. Next door was Martin's Hairdresser, 4 Prospect Street, and as I had my hair cut every four weeks it was useful, although I started going bald many years before. I even recall asking my doctor when I was 18 about treatment and he ducked his head and said, "Do you think I would be like this if I could grow hair on your head?"

Mr Martin told me he had cured three men of baldness. First he drew the skin right off the bald patch, then applied a lotion three times a day for 14 days while keeping the wound open. The lotion, which I think included vinegar and paraffin, had a horrible smell. It could not be packaged because it had a shelf life of only 14 days (which could have been due to the white of an egg) but he said it was successful.

William Avery, Pangbourne

Help from the cows

When I was a district nurse, one of my patients said her husband put half an onion under the bed to cure baldness. A farmer I knew swore that when he bent down to milk the cows they licked the top of his bald head and the saliva helped his hair to grow.

Mollie Smith

Japanese hint

Seaweed is good for you. The Japanese believe that it is particularly beneficial for the hair and will make it grow faster. Pregnant women eat seaweed so that their children will get nice black hair.

To make your hair grow thicker, cut it only when the moon is waxing. To make it grow longer, cut it when the moon is waning.

Foul with powdering

'Had Sarah to comb my head clean, which I find so foul with powdering and other troubles, that I am resolved to try how I can keep my head dry without powder; and I did also in a sudden fit cut off all my beard, which I have been a great while bringing up, only that I may with my pumice stone do my whole face, as I now do my chin, and so save time, which I find a very easy way, and gentle. She also washed my feet in a bath of herbs; and so to bed.'

Samuel Pepys, May 31, 1662

Disguising grey hair

To disguise grey hairs, rinse your hair with cold tea after shampooing. Another method is to mix one-sixth of an ounce of iron sulphate with nine ounces of red wine. Every morning, dip your comb in the mixture several times while combing your hair for five to ten minutes.

Mix five tablespoons of eucalyptus oil, four tablespoons of bay rum and one tablespoon of glycerine to rub into the hair.

Aunt Emily's recipes

Head

Recipe for headaches (19th century)

For a nervous headache, make a strong tea of common sage, with a little cayenne pepper. Sweeten and drink while warm. You can also use red sage, rosemary, and cayenne.

For a bilious headache, mix seven ounces senna, a quarter ounce sage, a quarter ounce ginger in one pint of boiling water. Drink one wine glass three times a day.

North American Indians and the first settlers used meadowsweet or Spiraea for relieving headaches and fevers. Now we know it contains salicin, which is aspirin, and is also found in poplars and willows.

Henna for the head

In Iraq, if you have a headache you dry henna leaves in the sun for half an hour, then mix them with tea and put it on your head. It cools you down.

Ahood Al-Rehani

Zimbabweans will cut a potato in half and strap it on their head if they have a headache. They think the poison goes into the potato turning it black.

Jack Callow

'The mind creates sickness'

Some Japanese remedies

We are very health conscious in Japan. Every day on Japanese lunch time television you will find health hints programmes when they talk about the importance of eating a healthy diet with a lot of vegetables, and fibre. They say that you need to eat 36 kinds of food each day to keep you healthy so it is very hard work to make balanced meals, and you need lots of little helpings. Fortunately we have a much wider variety of vegetables than in England.

English food is very greasy, with huge piles of chips. In Japan you would get a small pile of dry chips and eat the fish separately. Fish is very expensive now in Japan because of the polluted fishing waters. It used to be a common snack.

Fish with a shiny skin like mackerel and sardines are very healthy because they are low in cholesterol. Eel is good for you particularly in the summer and if you eat it you will survive the heat. It is full of Vitamin A.

We grill dried sardines and eat them from head to tail including the bones, which are full of calcium for your bones and teeth. Very fresh raw liver is good for the blood but of course you would never eat raw liver in the UK.

We use the water in which rice has been cooked, because it's good for your skin, and also useful for feeding plants, and some people say spinach can help your eyesight.

We have many cold cures. We make a drink of spring onions chopped and ground with a soya bean paste mixed with hot water, and we also drink honey, lemons and ginger. Japanese pumpkins are smaller and sweeter than the ones here, full of Vitamin C, and we eat them to keep away colds.

If you heat up Japanese saké mixed with raw egg it will warm you up, clear a blocked nose and soothe a headache. If you put saké in the bath, it is also good for the skin. We have a fruit called yuzu, a cross between a lime and an orange, which we put in the bath water. The day that winter begins, you bathe in water with yuzu juice in it and then you won't get colds.

In old times in winter, children took off their clothes, stripped to their underwear and rubbed their skin with a rough towel to keep warm.

We say, as you do in England, an apple a day keeps the doctor away. Japanese apples are huge but Japanese plums are small, sour and salty. You can't get them in England so we bring them with us, either dried or pickled. You can mix them with water or eat them with rice. If you drink plums in hot water a few times a day, it will stop diarrhoea.

We take aloe, cut up small, for stomach pains. It is also good for cold sores and ulcers, will cool sunburn, help circulation and get rid of chilblains.

We believe in the importance of pressure points which correspond to different parts of the body. You can see maps of these various points hanging in public baths and health centres. If you have sore eyes or a pain in the shoulder, hold the skin between

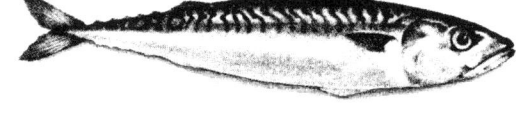

Healthy fish (from top): sardine, mackerel and eel

your thumb and forefinger. If it feels sore and hot, press it gently and you will feel better,

On the sole of your foot are pressure points which correspond to your organs. If you cut a piece of bamboo in half and step on it, it will find the pressure points and help tired feet and legs.

Some people believe if you have a spot or a pimple, you can visit a statue of a Buddha or a god, where incense is burning, take the ash from the incense stick, rub it on the skin and the spot will go.

People also go to temples and shrines where there is a statue of a saint and if any part of you hurts, you waft the smoke over the bad part.

It gets very hot and humid in Japan in the summer and in the days before air-conditioning the old-style house with wooden doors and paper screens allowed the building to breathe, and the air to circulate. Some country homes had gaps beneath the house to allow the air to circulate. In modern apartment blocks, they rely on air-conditioning.

In the garden, the Japanese will build a little waterfall so that the sound of running water will make you feel cool. In traditional Japanese sweetshops, teashops and restaurants you will find water dripping from a sort of bamboo see-saw and the sound of the water and the bamboo rubbing against bamboo is very refreshing.

Sumo

There is a Japanese proverb which says that the mind creates sickness. Before you take part in a sport such as kendo or sumo, or any kind of exercise, you practise mokusou – sit and close your eyes and clear your mind of all thoughts.

*Eiko, Sachiko, Yoko, and Yoshie
from the Gyosei College, Reading*

Eyes

Training the muscles

In South Africa if someone was short-sighted they were encouraged to immerse their face in a bowl of cold water and open their eyes. The water was supposed to have a therapeutic effect on the muscles which control the eyeballs.

Not long ago, I met a young man from Zambia who told me that he had started wearing glasses as a child and his grandmother had made him carry out this underwater exercise every day. He hasn't worn glasses since.

Rose Cam

The way to better sight

To improve my eyesight my ears were pierced before I was six months old according to the belief in Italy.

So why am I short sighted with an astigmatism?

Linda Maestranzi

For sore, tired eyes

If your eyes are tired with black circles underneath, boil some cornflowers in water. Allow them to cool then make compresses by putting the flowers between layers of gauze. Lie flat for 15 minutes with a compress over each eye.

Apply a raw potato cut in rounds each morning and evening to soothe swollen eyelids.

Ala Zolkiewka from Poland

Clean sore or infected eyes with cooled boiled salted water. Wipe inwards and down toward the nose using a different cotton wool ball for each wipe.

Egyptian artistry

The ancient Egyptians made black eye make-up

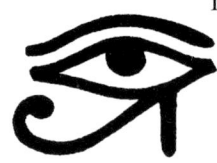

from galena, a native ore from which lead is obtained, and carbon scraped from above their fireplaces, mixed with goose fat. For green eye shadow they used powdered, emerald-green copper ore. These not only served as an adornment but protected the eyes from the numerous infectious eye diseases of Egypt.

The 'all-seeing' sacred eye of the Egyptian sun god Ra

'The nervous optick tremors came on in the evening, and a cup of beer helped, even on this my usual half-fast day.'

Dr John Rutty (1698-1774), doctor and diarist

To cure a stye (1907)

Put the smallest quantity of water possible over half a teaspoonful of black tea and allow it to steep.

After ten minutes fold the wet tea-leaves into a tiny piece of thin muslin. Lay it on the eyelid and keep the eyes shut for half an hour. This cure is only good before the stye has come to a head; the poultice must be applied as soon as the first prickling pain in the eyelid announces the inflammation.

Dandelion tea is reputed by Romanies to cure styes and conjunctivitis.

A salve of honey and cornmeal for pig-sties [sic].

17th century North American prescritpion

The evil eye

An ancient belief in Greece attributes magical power to the human eye. A shepherd whose sheep died one after the other could find no natural explanation. He feared that he had the evil eye and putting his fearful theory to the test, closed one eye and looked at the sheep. Nothing happened. He closed the other, looked again and one sheep died. Knowing he had an evil eye he tore it out.

Nosing around

For a nose bleed, make the patient stand erect, with arms raised above the head, bathe the face, douching it with iced water, put a small ice bag on the bridge of the nose, and on the nape of the neck.

Gently inhale through the bleeding nostril. Do not blow the nose. Cold to the nape of the neck and a hot mustard and water footbath may be tried. Firmly nipping the nostrils with finger and thumb stops the bleeding.

The R.E.P. Book (1903)

A physician in ancient Egypt advised that bandages should be stuffed into the nostrils to stop nosebleeds. "That does hinder the breathing, but the flow of blood is stopped."

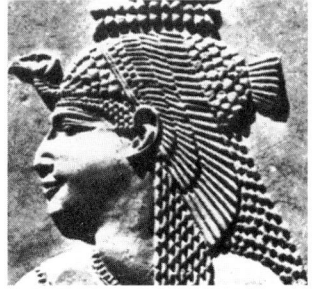

Hildegard's theory

A German 12th century mystic healer, Hildegard of Bingen, had her own explanation for sneezing.

Whenever the blood in the vessels goes to sleep and other fluids become lazy, she said, the soul notices this and causes the body to tremble through sneezing. This wakes up the blood and juices of the person so that they become awake and lively.

Ears

A burning sensation

This is an Italian cure
for earaches caused by
excess wax. Melt beeswax
and spread it over a
small piece of linen.
As it hardens, roll
the linen into a thin
tube. Place into the ear
and light the top. (You need help for this!) Allow it
to burn slowly halfway down.

It seems that as the wax burns, a vacuum forms
and sucks out any hard wax from the ear canal
which then collects in the bottom part of the linen
tube. It really works and is much less painful than
being syringed. Just take care not to catch fire!

The normal remedy is to warm some olive oil on a
teaspoon and pour a few drop into the ear canal.
Plug with cotton wool. This will soothe and soften
the wax and should work on minor cases.

Some people suggest squeezing the contents from
a garlic capsule into the ear.

....

**A gipsy remedy from Berkshire for earache is a
roast onion placed on the ear.**

....

Lemon juice is a powerful bactericide so if you have
an earache squeeze a few drops of juice on to some
warmed cotton wool and plug the ear with it.

A cure for deafness or slow hearing

The juice of radishes, the fat of mole, an eel and the
juice of onion, all soaked in wine and roasted. Boys'
urine is also good.

17th century New England remedies

The smell of geraniums

If we had ear infections and the ear was not open-
ing up to drain, my South African grandmother
twisted a leaf of a geranium between her fingers and
put it on the outside of the ear. The smell of the
geranium had some potent effect and the infections
would be drawn out with no ill effects.

Rose Cam

Just carelessness

from The Daily Mail (July 11, 1896)

Many deformities, which it is impossi-
ble to remedy in adults, are the result
of the carelessness or thoughtlessness
of nurses and mothers. The simple
matter of a shapely or unshapely ear
may be settled in infancy if a little
attention be given by those who have
the baby's good looks, as well as health,
in their keeping.

If the infant's ears show a mulish tendency to
stand out from the head, something should be done
about it, especially if the child be a boy. Caps can be
purchased for the purpose of confining too prominent ears and keeping them close to the head. They
are rather expensive, but one that will answer the
purpose can be made at home. Take a strip of
muslin about three inches wide, pass it over the
ears, and cut it the right length to meet beneath the
chin; fasten a band to it to cross the back of the
head, another at the nape of the neck, and a third
across the forehead.

Tie the cap with strings under the chin; it is
intended to be worn at night. Prominent ears are
sometimes due to an over-development of cartilage
at the back of the ear, and this can be remedied
only by a surgical operation.

Mouth

Advice for nurse

When I was a district nurse, one of my elderly patients noticed I had a cold sore on my lip. "You know what you need for that – earhole grease," she said. You had to rub your finger behind your ear and apply it on the sore. I didn't try it.

Mollie Smith

....
An old Wiltshire lip salve was hog's lard washed in rose-water.
....

A naval cure for gumboils

A gumboil is usually caused by a stump or decayed tooth. The pain is very severe, especially at night. A raisin baked hot in the oven, split in two, and the inside part, free from seeds, placed upon the painful spot will, acting as a poultice, ease the pain and bring the swelling to a head, when it should be lanced with the point of an abscess knife directed towards the bone; instant relief will follow.

The Ship Captain's Medical Guide (1912)

Teeth

Sparkling smile

Pakistani women clean their teeth with the special bark of a tree, dan da sa. It makes your teeth sparkle, your mouth tingle and your teeth feel smooth. You rub your teeth for four or five minutes to get the full brightness. You can chew the bark to help with toothache, and it brings the colour to your lips if you haven't lipstick.

Akhtar Aziz

For decayed gums

Add powdered grapevine ash to a good wine and brush your teeth often.

Hildegard of Bingen, 12th century mystic healer

....

For the teeth: Port Wine – a quarter of a pint; Vinegar – a quarter of a pint; Brandy – a wine glass; Myrrh – an ounce, either powder or tincture; Salt – an handful; Water – as much as will make the whole quantity a pint.

18th century receipt

....

Alum and cloves

An old remedy for toothache is putting a pinch of alum or a small piece of clove on the tooth.

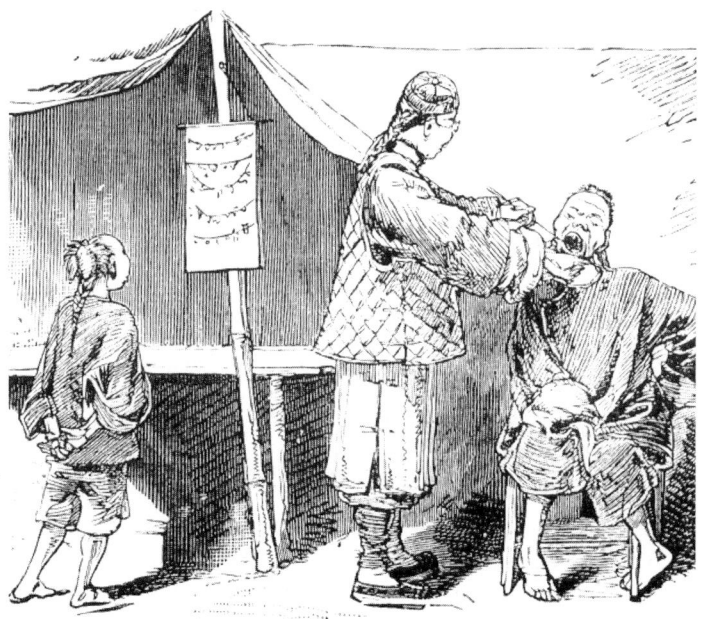

A Chinese street tooth-drawer at his stall extracting a tooth from a patient   Wellcome Institute Library, London

Vinegar and brown paper...

In north-west Leicestershire, toothache was treated by applying brown paper which had been soaked in vinegar and sprinkled with pepper. This was held in place by a scarf.

Before 1900, dentists could not be found in the poorer parts of the Midlands and a bad tooth meant a visit to the local blacksmith who had special pincers for teeth. Many blacksmiths became very skilled at making a quick extraction.

Tony Barham

...and again

Face-ache (neuralgia) is often caused by a decayed and hollow tooth. If badly decayed, extraction is the only permanent shipboard remedy. If the pain is very intense, a mustard-leaf or a piece of brown paper dipped in vinegar and well peppered may be put on the side of the face and kept in position by a large handkerchief.

The Ship Captain's Medical Guide
(1912)

Charcoal for teeth

We would use charcoal to clean our teeth in South Africa. My dad never used a toothbrush because he believed they wore the gums down and made your teeth longer. We would burn coal and keep charcoal in lumps in a container and every morning we would grind them down to a powder and brush our teeth. We used twigs like an orange stick and our teeth were impeccable.

Rose Cam

The mind

Sonning pilgrims

Pilgrims on a visit to Hambleden would sometimes make a diversion to visit a well not far from Bisham Abbey which was considered good for sore or infected eyes. Those who were prepared to venture further upstream could seek out the Chapel of Saint Cyrick at Sonning, where there had been miraculous cures of people suffering from mental illness.

A short distance above Sonning they could visit Marian's Chapel, close to Caversham Bridge, where an extraordinary collection of miracle-working relics was kept.

'Witchcraft in the Thames Valley' Tony Barham

Nineteenth century Dartmoor gypsies believed that a stew or soup made from hedgehog could benefit the mentally afflicted.

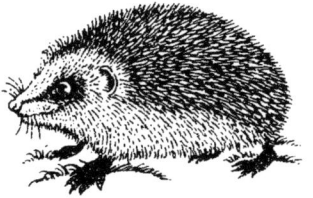

For Lunacy

'Take three handfuls of fresh Ground Ivy. Do not wash but rub it clean then put it into a piece of holland rag and Pound in a Marble Mortar. This should produce three Tablespoonfuls of Juice. Let the Patient take it nine mornings fasting with an Asafoetida Pill every night to strengthen the nerves then Drop it for nine mornings and then take it again.

'Lady Huntingdon gave it in fifty nine cases and it was never know[n] to fail if strictly attended to.'

Extract from the Revd Samuel Eyles Pierce letters (1809)

Boreline in the head

People who suffered from a mental illness in South Africa would have a boreline drilled in their head by an elder.

Rose Cam

Insomnia

Gentle sleep

Infusions containing *Valeriana radix* (valerian), *Melissa officinalis*(lemon balm) and *Mentha piperita* (peppermint) herbs have been consumed by insomniacs in Moravia for many years.

Moy Trchalik

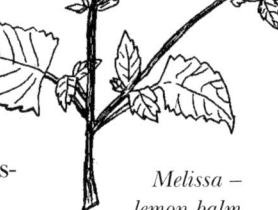

Melissa – lemon balm

Mother Jame, a 19th century wise-woman, prescribed raw onions for as a remedy for insomnia and sleep disorders.

Sleep on a hop-filled pillow

Chamomile tea is used in Italy for nearly everything, especially stress, insomnia and indigestion. Infuse in a covered cupful of boiling water.

Apply a hard-boiled egg to the nape of the neck peeled.

Dr John Perkins of Boston, USA, 18th century

In mild cases an infusion of Ladies' Slipper, chamomile, hops and wild lettuce is often sufficient.

'Get Back to Nature and Live' CW Aloysius Browne

An oil for all purposes

Tea-Tree Oil has been used safely in its native Australia for over seventy years but it was known long before then by Aborigines who used the tea-tree as a herbal remedy for centuries. They chewed young leaves for sore throats, inhaled it for chest problems, macerated it and used it as poultices and they knew the oil kept away insects and acted as an antiseptic.

Melaleuca alternifolia or tea-tree, the source of the medicinal tea-tree oil, is an evergreen found in Queensland and on the north coast of Northern New South Wales. It is six metres high with a four metre spread, and its stem is erect, smooth and bushy with papery bark. The flowers, which bloom from spring to early summer, are white in dense terminal heads.

Tea-tree oil contains at least 48 known organic compounds. It is a germicide and also helps relieve pain since it has a mild, local anaesthetic action.

It is a strong organic solvent, penetrating deeply through the skin, even reaching under the finger nails into boils and sores, dissolving the pus, but is soothing on application.

It kills bacteria fast and effectively without damaging healthy cells, and destroys many fungal organisms which cause skin problems.

Recommended as a shampoo, tea-tree oil is a natural cleanser assisting in the treatment of dandruff and other scalp conditions, while acting as a tonic on the scalp. It is used as part of a tea-tree oil head-lice treatment.

Tea-tree oil kills the bacteria which produce the odour in perspiration without stopping perspiration which is much safer than aluminum-based deodorants.

An antiseptic cream containing five per cent tea-tree oil will soothe bites, rashes, chicken pox, sores, nappy rash, and dermatitis, and can even be massaged into sore joints to relieve the pain.

It is recommended for pimples, abrasions, athletes foot, cuts and minor burns, to name but a few of its applications. This is especially useful for diabetics who are at greater risk of developing fungal infections.

Further diluted, the oil can be spread over a large area of skin with a minimum risk of irritation.

Many other tea-tree products are available but worth mentioning are the throat lozenges, which contain a mixture of herbs and dried tea-tree leaf, and tea-tree toothpaste.

Tea-tree oil as well as being a bactericide and fungicide has also been found effective against the wart virus both plantar and regular. A recipe for warts consists of two teaspoons of tea-tree oil with three tablespoons of tree of life tincture. Shake well then apply one or two drops of the mixture up to four times a day.

For a healing mixture, use one part of tea-tree oil diluted with eight parts of calendula and apply to the skin. For acne, steam the face with two drops each of lavender, camomile and tea-tree oil added to hot water.

Margaret Skinner

Tea-tree – Melaleuca quinquenervia

Important: If you are using tea-tree oil for the first time it is wise to test a small patch on the underside of the arms. If any redness or skin irritation develops or persists after using then discontinue its use and the skin will recover. Never apply undiluted oil to the skin and keep out of the reach of children.

Neck Lines

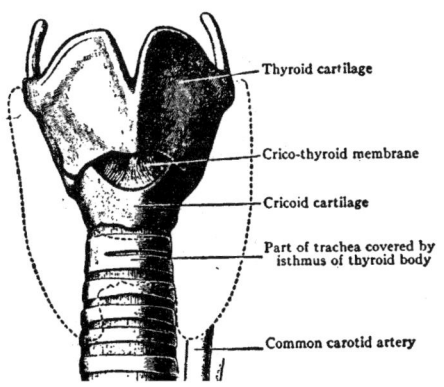

Thyroid cartilage

Crico-thyroid membrane

Cricoid cartilage

Part of trachea covered by
isthmus of thyroid body

Common carotid artery

*'Keene's One Night Cold
Cure will break up any
cold overnight; or money
refunded! Influenza cured in three
days. Guarantee label around
every Box.'*

Advertisement c 1909

Throat

Coughs and colds

Queen Victoria's remedy

Before 1948 and the start of the National Health Service, with its promise of medical care from the cradle to the grave, more people resorted to home remedies and herbal cures. These restoratives varied in efficacy and many entered the folklore surrounding the subject and are referred to as old wives' tales.

In most communities there existed someone who had acquired knowledge of plant materials, usually known as the 'wise woman', because in the main this practice came from women. One such lady lived in our road in Ireland. She attended births, nursed the sick and laid out the dead. A large, formidable character, with hair drawn back into a severe bun, she was nicknamed Queen Victoria by us children. She dispensed potions, ointments and medicines from her dark cottage with its smoke-stained walls.

My sister and I had developed persistent irritating coughs which the usual lemon and honey had failed to remove. My mother had decided to consult Queen Victoria and returned home with instructions on how to make an efficacious remedy. As I remember it, the main ingredients were black treacle and a pennyworth of 'all fours' (liquorice, aniseed, ipecacuanha and peppermint).

These were mixed with water and set on the side of the range where it bubbled merrily almost smiling at us, but masking its malevolence. We tasted it while still warm and found it quite pleasant but when it was cold there was a complete transformation, the taste became revolting. Whether it was the fuss my sister and I created at the disgusting taste, the length of time preparing the concoction, or the sticky mess of the saucepan when it had to be cleaned, my mother never gave us any more of Queen Victoria's remedy.

Roisin O'Callaghan

Cough mixtures

A home-made remedy

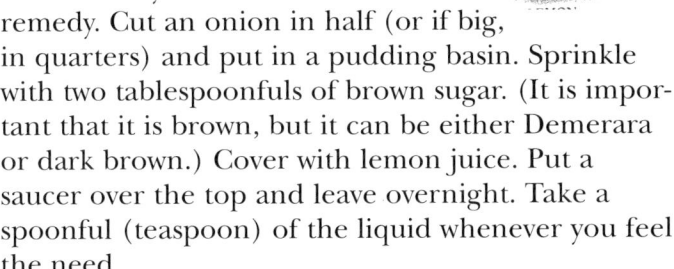

If you have a tickly, dry cough, forget commercial cough mixtures and try this home-made remedy. Cut an onion in half (or if big, in quarters) and put in a pudding basin. Sprinkle with two tablespoonfuls of brown sugar. (It is important that it is brown, but it can be either Demerara or dark brown.) Cover with lemon juice. Put a saucer over the top and leave overnight. Take a spoonful (teaspoon) of the liquid whenever you feel the need.

You can't overdose and it won't make you drowsy. If you have a chesty cough that persists for more than a week, see your doctor as you may have an infection that needs more than cough mixture.

Betty O'Rourke

Mix brandy, hot water, raw egg and honey. It's disgusting but it soothes your throat.

Ahood Al-Rehani from Iraq

Five ounces honey, four ounces treacle, half a pint of vinegar. Simmer for 15 minutes. When cool add three teaspoonsful of ipecacuanha wine. Take two teaspoons every four hours.

Vinegar and treacle

Half a pint of vinegar, half a pound of black treacle (Fowlers), two drachms each of laudanum, linseed, paregoric, syrup of squills, ipecacuanha. Put vinegar into a china saucepan, make it hot, dissolve the treacle in it and the other ingredients. Bottle and keep well corked.

Dose: dessertspoonful in water for adults, cold water during day, warm water at night.

Aunt Emily's recipe

....

Rub chests with camphorated oil and suck a sugar knob soaked in Friar's Balsam before retiring each night. Eucalyptus inhaled on a handkerchief should clear the nasal passages.

....

Cakes and ale

An ancient Mesopotamian (Iraqi) prescription against coughing: "Grind up sunflower in fine beer, honey, and purified oil and let the patient's tongue seize it without his tasting it and swallow the water of it. Give him beer and honey to drink cold, then with a wing feather make him vomit. Now the patient ought to eat bread or cake with cream and honey and drink sweet wine."

Colds

Five ways to cure a cold (1907)

1 Bathe the feet in hot water, and drink a pint of hot lemonade. Then sponge with salt water, and remain in a warm room.
2 Bathe the face in very hot water every five minutes for an hour.
3 Snuff hot salt water up the nostrils every three hours.
4 Inhale ammonia or menthol.
5 Take four hours' active exercise in the open air.

More cold remedies

A glass of hot wine with nine drops of beeswax, to be taken before bed.

17th century New England remedy

....

A Lemon or Two, clarified Honey (clarified first), and Sweet oil, simmered together. Also for a cold: Linseed and stick Liquorish made into Tea.

From Mary Loder's recipe book (18th century)

....

Put a few drops of eucalyptus oil in a bowl of hot water, bend over it with a towel over your head and inhale it.

Marguerite Hudson from Australia

Africans will crush eucalyptus leaves and sniff them to clear their sinuses.

Jack Callow, Zimbabwe

Rhubarb and sweet nitre

My mother used to send me to the chemist to buy tincture of rhubarb and sweet nitre. We took this with sugar in hot water (as hot as possible) for colds.

Marjorie Pemble

Onion juice and salt

We never went to a doctor when we were children in Italy. Mum would fill a bag with salt and tie it around our necks though I can't remember what for – a cold I think. She would rub Vick or some other strong-smelling ointment on our chests and wrap a flannel around our necks.

We would also cook up a lot of onions and drink the juice. The house would smell for days!

Teresa Mortl

A tot of rum

My Austrian great uncle who died at 97 (that was only because his calor gas cooker leaked) swore that the reason he never caught a cold was because he drank a small tot of rum every morning.

Linda Maestranzi

We didn't rush to the doctor so much in Sumatra. Ginger and lemongrass, crushed and boiled in water with dark brown sugar, strained and kept in a jar, is good for indigestion and colds and coughs. Fennel and green cardamom tea with two or three cloves added is good for a runny nose or as a refreshing drink instead of tea or coffee.

Dalip Chand

Horehound and hyssop

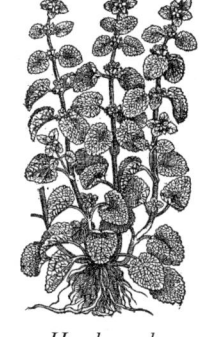

For a violent Cold and Cough horehound, hyssop and ground ivy, a handful of each, a stick of liquorice. Boil these gently in two quarts of spring water, then strain and boil up a second time, adding half a pound of stoned raisins and half a pound of sliced figs, and one head of garlic. Boil it to reduce to a quart. When cold strain and bottle.

Horehound

Take two or three spoonsful night and morning.

For a Gargle: Handfull of Bryer Leaves, a handfull of Common Barley boild in a Pint and a half of Water till it comes to a Pint. Add two ounces of Honey, and two Spoonfulls of Vinegar.

From Mary Loder's recipe book (18th century)

Disinfectant and senna

Mother was scrupulously clean. They said that she was born with with a disinfectant can in her hand. She once had enteric fever and when she got better she disinfected the whole house. I remember during the great flu epidemic of 1918, when I was five years old, Mother used to hang towels soaked in pine disinfectant over the doors in our bedroom. It was a dreadful smell but no one from my family caught flu.

Once a week Mother dosed us with senna, whether you needed it or not. She didn't ask if you had been. Today they don't care if you don't go for a week. I think it was better then. We also were given cod liver oil and malt at school but I think our parents had to pay for it. You had to be practically dead to get anything free in those days.

Mother would knit us woolly stockings that went up to our knees – most inelegant but they kept us warm. For headaches she would place a cloth soaked in vinegar on our forehead.

We didn't seem to get ill like people do these days. Our food was wonderful. Beautiful potatoes, greens, sprouts, turnips, watercress every Sunday – a whole bunch for one penny. We didn't have any foreign vegetables. My father had an allotment and we had some kind of greens every day. We had liver once a week and a hot joint on Sunday, then cold on Monday.

My father always had a bag of walnuts in his pockets. He used to say they were very good for us. So did my husband. He believed in the goodness in seeds and he made me promise that I would always take vitamin E for the rest of my life after he died, and I do. Nowadays I take garlic tablets and cod liver oil tablets as well as vitamin E. I also eat a lot of celery in soups. It's a diuretic, good for arthritis and I eat a bunch a week.

When I was young we couldn't afford oranges but Mother gave us a hot lemon drink once a week to keep us free of colds. We also ate lots of blackcurrants and blackberries. Then, we could pick them off the roadside because there wasn't much pollution from cars. Tomatoes are very good for you and the more sun they get the better they are for you. We ate a lot of fresh bread – you bought it by weight in those days – and we drank cocoa before bedtime. Horlicks was too expensive.

You couldn't afford to be ill, you were too busy. We did a lot of walking because we had to. My father would walk five miles each morning to get milk.

You weren't allowed to stay away from school. Someone would come round to your house straight away if you did. I was once ill and had to to sit in the hall all day.

In the 1920s it cost three

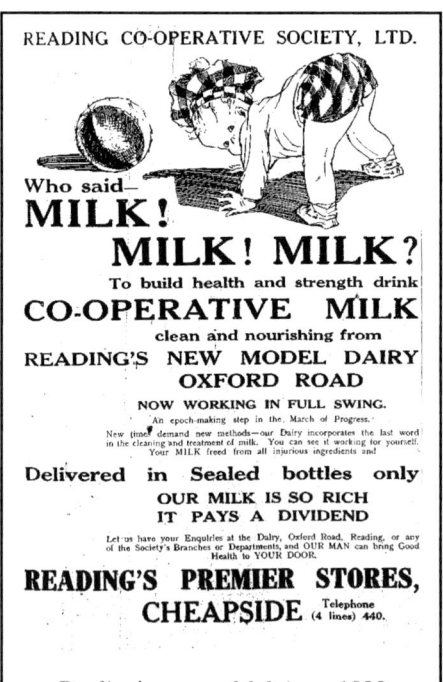

Reading's new model dairy – 1933

shillings and sixpence to see a doctor – an awful lot when you think that a man earned only £1 10 shillings a week on the railways. We would all go to the doctor's together and the well-to-do people there would look down on us. A nurse and a dentist would visit the schools.

The NHS made a big difference. In my day you went in to hospital to die. They didn't have all these operations you have today. I remember that if you got scarlet fever you were placed behind glass for weeks.

You had to pay to go into hospital to have a baby. When we gave birth we had to stay in bed for 14 days – we weren't allowed to get up, not like today. Now they say that staying in bed isn't good for you. If you had a bad time you had to stay even longer. I had a big baby and stayed 15 days. You were taught to feed your child because you couldn't afford to do otherwise. If you couldn't breastfeed, you bought National Milk.

When the next generation remembered that their neighbours had 20 children they only had one or two. I didn't have any choice about how many I had because the war came and I didn't want to bring another child into the world while that was on. After the war I could not have any more.

My husband had one leg and when I tried to get a downstairs council flat we were told that we didn't have enough points. I remember being asked if my husband had TB and I lost my temper and told them where to put their flat.

They were terrible days.

A Woodley pensioner

Sore throats

Croatian sugar

What everyone with a sore throat is looking for is instant relief. In Croatia we make a simple drink that does just that. All you need are three to four spoonsful of sugar and a cup of cold milk.

Melt the sugar in a pot and keep stirring until it becomes a nice, smooth, piping hot dark liquid, then pour in the milk. Stir a little and you will end up with big lumps of crystal sugar, which look and taste like sweets (I know I can never resist eating a couple of these). Wait until the milk boils, by which time the sugar will melt, then pour into a cup and drink it hot. It will not just soothe your throat, it is a very pleasant drink too.

Small children will love it, especially if you let them eat a couple of those 'sweets' before the sugar melts.

Silvia Kufner

....

If you had a sore throat you'd soak a sock in embrocation and wrap it round your neck.

Cyril Shuffle, aged 91

....

You'd tie tarred string round your sore throat – but it made your neck black.

George Pottinger, aged 88

Balm for a sore throat

Mix one ounce of marsh mallow root and one ounce of honey in four-fifths of a pint of water. Gargle well with the liquid several times a day, Alternatively, gargle with salt and water – half a teaspoon to a glass of water – or with the juice of a lemon in a glass of warm water.

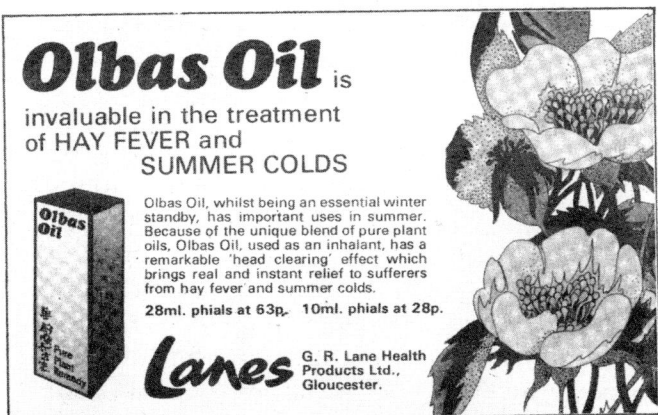

A 1960s advertisement from G R Lane Health Products

Garlic and ginger

My grandmother would break off a little chunk of
dried root ginger for us to chew for a sore throat.
She would also give us a liquid made from ginger
pounded up, sliced onion, very hot chilli sliced up,
garlic, lemon juice, and tomatoes. She would let it
stand for three days, then spoonfed us with this very
hot liquid. The sore throat would go in no time at
all because garlic and ginger are natural antibiotics.

Rose Cam

....

**For hoarseness: take a fresh egg, beat it and
thicken it with castor sugar; flavour it to taste with
lemon. Take promptly. (1907)**

....

Soot and alum

In Pakistan we have an old cure for tonsillitis. When
we make chapatties on a hot plate over the open
fire, soot collects on the bottom. We take this soot,
mix it with alum, wet it with the thumb, put it on
the finger, make the victim say "Aagh" and touch
the tonsils. After two or three doses, they recover.

Akhtar Aziz

Herbs, ancient and modern

Over the past few years there has been an upsurge of interest in old-time natural and herbal remedies which are now being recognised and used in up-to-date cures.

Many people wouldn't know a henbane from a hyssop, but everyone can recognise a daisy. It is said that nature made this plant common because it is so useful. It is sometimes used by homeopaths as a remedy for lumps and swellings caused by injury, and for skin diseases such as boils, among other things.

Hyssop

The wild poppy is easy enough to spot. The flowers can be made into a syrup to soothe a cough and induce sleep. An infusion of the petals may be helpful in treating chest complaints. The opium poppy contains morphine and codeine so, unless you know exactly what you are doing, it is safer to steer clear of home-made remedies!

Then there is dog's-grass, commonly known as couch-grass. How much energy have you spent in trying to evict it from your garden? Yet it is said to contain an antibiotic substance, is an ideal remedy for cystitis and has been found helpful to those with gout and rheumatism.

Nettles appear to have many uses too, though the idea of placing the bruised leaves up the nostrils to remove a polypus may not appeal to most people. However, nettle tea is highly recommended to arthritis sufferers and as a blood purifier. The young leaves picked (preferably while wearing thick gloves) and boiled in a little water make a passable substitute for spinach. Many country folk used this during the last war to supplement their vitamins.

The sophisticated orchid also has its country cousin. At one time the dried root was powdered and made into a nourishing drink. Witches are said to have administered it for its aphrodisiac properties. At a more down-to-earth level it was claimed to 'kill worms in children'.

Dried sage leaves infused in boiling water and used as a gargle are very soothing to sore throats and safe enough to use for oneself.

A strong decoction of the wild pansy is claimed to be an excellent cure for venereal diseases. Its modern uses are stated as being 'mildly laxative, diuretic, diaphoretic and expectorant'. Any wonder that it is also known as heart's-ease?

Wild pansies

Ever used a dock leaf to relieve a nettle sting? But did you know that if you boil dock leaves with meat it will make it 'boil the sooner'? Perhaps unnecessary in these days of the microwave.

Arssmart, a member of the polygonum family, would appear to be a most versatile plant. It is effective for 'putrid ulcers and destroys worms in the ears'. Not only that but if it be 'strewn about the floor of the chamber it will soon kill all the fleas'. If you have a tired horse, put a good handful of this under the saddle, it will make him travel better. One wonders what it can possibly contain.

There are herbs for everything from ague to warts. There are emetics, diuretics, potions to enhance one's sex life, lotions to curb it. The more that you learn of this subject the more you realise how little you know of it. Yet in bygone days every village had its crone who was conversant with all these cures.

Carol Whelan

Shivers and shakes

St Vitus dance

Local tradition in Wychwood Forest, Oxfordshire.
tells of a wise woman who came from time to time
to the forest in the 1850s to collect mould from
leaves and damp wood. She used this for a concoction to remedy St Vitus Dance.

'Witchcraft in the Thames Valley' Tony Barham

'Having had several violent fits of an ague, recourse
was had to bathing my legs in milk up to the knees,
made as hot as I could endure it; and sitting so in it
in a deep churn, or vessel, covered with blankets,
and drinking carduus posset [Blessed Thistle, used
as a posset-drink for fevers], then going to bed and
sweating, I not only missed that expected fit, but
had no more, only continued weak, that I could not
go to church till Ash-Wedneday, which I had not
missed, I think, so long in twenty years, so gracious
had God been to me.'
(February 7, 1682)

John Evelyn (1620-1706)

**'I took early in the morning a good dose
of Elixir and hung three spiders about
my neck and they drove my ague away.
Deo gratias.'**

Elias Ashmole (1617-92), antiquarian

As a child in Zimbabwe I used to think acacia
trees were called fever trees because they
grow near rivers and places where malaria is
prevalent. But in fact it is because they can cure
fever. The bark has a quinine-like substance in it
and can be boiled and drunk as a medicine.

Jack Callow

Skin Deep

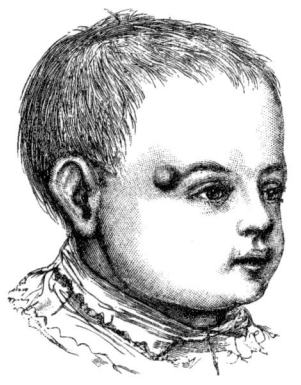

'*In the treatment of torturing, disfiguring, itching, scaly, crusted, pimply, blotchy and scrofulous humours of the skin, scalp, and blood, [these] remedies have been wonderfully successful.*'

Advertisement c 1907

Skin

Dog and snake bites

18th century Remedy for the biting of a Mad Dogg

This was found in the parish records of Sunninghill, followed by a note: NB This receipt was taken out of Calhorp [sic] Church in Lincolnshire, almost the whole town being Bitten with a Mad Dogg. All that took this Medicine did live and those others Died Mad.

Take the Leaves of Rue picked from the Stalks and Bruised Six Ounces, Garlick pick'd from the Stalks and Bruised, Venice Treacle or Mithridats, and the Scrapings of Pewtor of each 6 Ounces. Boil all this over a Slow fire, in Two Quarts of Strong Ale; till one Pint be confined; Then stop it in a botle clost Stopt, and give of it 9 Spoon fulls to a Man or Woman Warm, Seven Mornings together fasting, and Six for a Dogg.
This the Author believing will not (by God's Blessing) fail if it be given within 9 days after the biting of the Dogg. Apply Some of the Ingredients from which the Liquor was strained to the bitten place.

An Infallible cure for the Bite of a mad dog

This medicine has been given to hundreds with success and Sir George Cobb has cured two people with the Symptoms of madness upon them.
24 grains of natural cinnabar and 24 grains of fictitious cinnabar and 16 grains of musk ground together finely, put in a small tea cup of rum or

brandy and mixed well. To be given to the patient as soon as possible after the bite, and then again 30 days later. But if the symptoms of madness occur, to give a dose immediately and another an hour later.

The Benyon family of Englefield (18th and 19th century)

Against ye bite of Serpents and Vipers

Imprimo: Whilst ye remedy is preparing ye must, if possible, tightly bind ye pte above ye wound to prevent ye progress of ye venom.

2dly: With ye assistance of any sharp instrument, make a small incision on ye wound, which will yield a few drops of water; then burn ye wound 3 or 4 times. Dip a bit of Linen Rag within Hungary Water, and set it near enough to a light that it may catch fire, and let ye flame touch ye wound.

3dly: Apply to ye wound a Plaister made of the best Venice Treacle, mixed with a large pinch of powder of Vipers, and an equal quantity of Oyster Shell calcified and pulverised, apply it to ye wound; change this within 2 days, and let a fresh plaister to be put on ye venom, 4 or 5 days, taking great care not to wet ye afflicted part as long as ye Plaister continues on ye wound. On account of ye sweat which will be occasioned by ye bites, ye plaister must be covered well with ye Treacle and Ingredients 2 or 3 times a day.

4thly: After ye foregoing preparations, let ye patient for 3 or 4 days take ye same as a tincture diluted in red or white wine, observing to take y^e dose in a Morning fasting, and not to eat or drink any thing for two hours after. The dose must be proportionally less for Children.

From Wallingford Borough Records, dated 1785, and
believed to originate from the parish of Thame

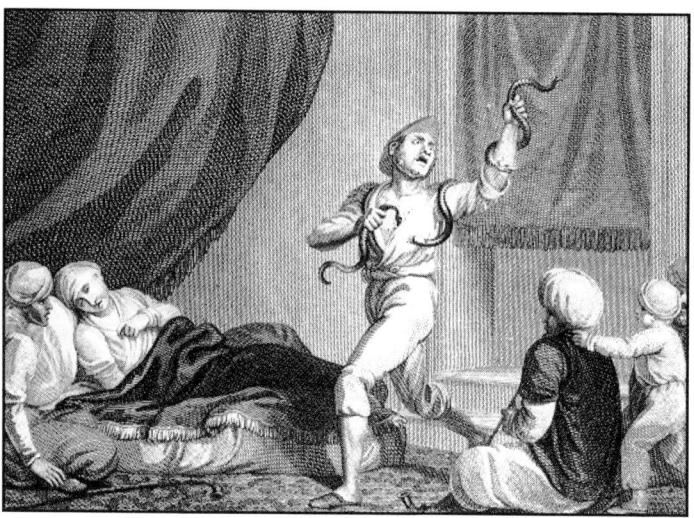

A Saadi, or Egyptian shaman, using snakes and incantations to cure a sick man

Wellcome Institute Library, London

Snakes in the bed

In South Africa, garlic was used as snake deterrent. People would plant garlic plants outside the door and the snakes did not seem to like them. Without garlic, you got something slithery in your bed!

Rose Cam

....

The leaf of plantain as a poultice laid to the part bitten immediately fetches out the deadly poison. It is also remarkable that if put into the shoes, no serpent will dare to come near them.

17th century New England remedy

....

Boils

If you had a boil, the custom in Southern Italy was to cut a tomato and place it over the boil to bring it out. Tomato purée was also used on burns.

Teresa Mortl

This is an old remedy for boils or any festering wound from which poisons need to be extracted: put some bread in a piece of muslin and pour boiling water over it. Squeeze out surplus water and apply the poultice on the boil straight away.

Marjorie Pemble

To make black Salve

Good for everything particularly Boils

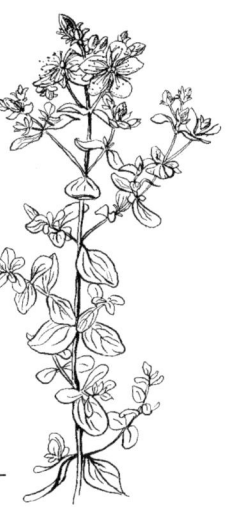

St John's Wort

Half a Pound of Red Lead beaten or sifted well or fine; two ounces of Castrel [sic] Soap; two Ounces of Bees Wax; one Ounce of Oyl of Saint Johns Wort; one Pint of Oyl of Olive; put the Pint of Oyl into a little Pot, and cut the Soap and Wax into it, then let it boil till the Soap and Wax are all melted, then put in the Oyl of St Johns Wort and let it boil a little, then take it off the fire and stir in the Red Lead, then boil it all together till it begins to grow black; your pot must not be above half full; then pour it into a Pan of Cold Water and when you can, roll it up.

From Mary Loder's recipe book (18th century)

Boils at sea

A simple remedy for boils and also a preventive, is a couple of teaspoonsful of flour in a small cup of cold water taken upon an empty stomach in the early morning. When the boils show a tendency to form or are in actual progress, the bowels should be kept active by giving a teaspoonful of Epsom salts mixed in a tumbler full of the ordinary ship's lime juice and water; half a pint should be given twice daily.

Do not treat boils with the favourite soap and sugar application, and avoid linseed poultices, which afford the surest way of raising a crop of them when they once threaten to appear.

The skin should be first well cleaned all round the affected surface with lint dipped in Spirit of Ammonia or Turpentine, and then covered with Boric lint wrung out in hot water; the skin must be handled and touched as little as possible. When matter is forming, a match dipped in pure Carbolic acid should be used to drill a small hole in the to allow the core to escape.

The Ship Captain's Medical Guide (1912)

Ancient Egyptians recognised the medicinal benefits of yeast (which contains vitamin B and antibiotic agents) which they applied raw to ulcers and boils and took for digestive disorders.

Bruises

Tincture of arnica painted on knocks to bones brings out bruises.

Gladys Bradford

Butter brings out a bruise after a fall.

To relieve a bruise and sprain, dissolve a teaspoon of camphor in half a pint of olive oil to make a liniment. Rub in twice a day.

Burns

In Australia, we use Aloe Vera, a fleshy cactus-like plant with soft spikes, for burns. Peel back the green skin and press the white flesh on the burn. When you have eaten a slice of water-melon, wipe the skin over your shoulders and arms to ease sunburn.

Marguerite Hudson

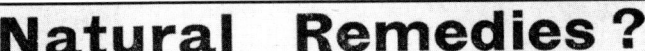

Quiet Life tablets – from an 1980s advertisement for G R Lane Health Products Limited

For a burn (1907)

The white of an egg applied to a scald or burn is most soothing, and will heal it quickly.

....

Cold water and oatmeal used as a poultice will relieve burns, or cloths soaked in cold water. Keep the air away and, as soon as you can, dress it with Herbal Unguentum or Olive Oil.

'Get Back to Nature and Live' C W Aloysius Browne

....

Potato poultice (c 1920s)

For a minor burn, if there is no broken skin, rub the burn with a slice of raw potato. A potato poul-tice will give rapid relief from sunburn. Grate raw potato and spread between two layers of gauze. Apply this to the face or other affected parts.

Cool burnt skin with yogurt or tomato purée.

Ahood Al-Rehani

A Spanish remedy for sunburn – a flannel soaked in vinegar and laid on sunburn cools and soothes.

Trini Bello

If a baby got burned in South Africa, someone would quickly pee on the area which was affected.

Cold tea

Cold tea-leaves, bound on a burn, take the fire out at once. When there is no cold tea in the house, pour boiling water on tea-leaves, let it stand for a moment, drain, squeeze through cold water, and apply to the burn.

Cuts

Guava leaves

Philippinos use the fresh young leaves of the guava plant boiled in water to treat cuts. This is used mainly to help circumcision wounds heal faster.

Lani Barwick

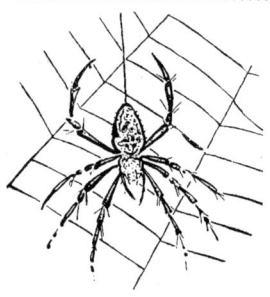

One old lady told me her grandma kept a cupboard full of cobwebs in case a child fell and cut their knees. Cobwebs on the wound were meant to help the blood clot so that it healed quickly.

Mollie Smith

Drawing infection

The datura plant, which spreads like wildfire in South Africa, is used for drawing infection from wounds. Because it is poisonous you cannot put it directly on to skin, but you wrap it in a cloth and the heat draws it out.

Battle scars

At the battle of Agincourt (1415) soldiers would urinate on the wounds. It acted as an antiseptic.

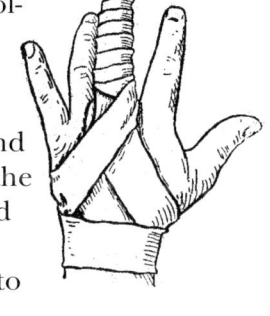

Penobscot Indians from New England still scrape the gum off the bark of the balsam fir to cover and heal cuts and burns, and, during battles, Maine Indians used the gummy substance to clean wounds.

....

Herb Robert, also called Adder's Tongue, Death Come Quickly, and Poor Robert, is said to be useful in stopping the bleeding of wounds.

....

Early Indian surgeons used large black Bengali ants to help suture intestinal wounds. The ants' mandibles clamped the edges of the wound and these were left behind when the heads were separated from the bodies and left in the intestines.

Bushman's Friend

The leaves of the New Zealand rangiora plant contain a poisonous but antiseptic property which can be applied to wounds. This useful plant is familiarly known as the Bushman's Friend because the leaves can be used as a substitute for toilet paper. A poultice made by boiling the leaves of another plant, the kawakawa, helps to heal infected wounds.

Eczema

Berkshire gypsies believed you should bathe in sea water to cure eczema. Dartmoor gypsies recommend milk or cream from a red cow for this and various other skin conditions.

Tony Barham

Ancient moisturiser

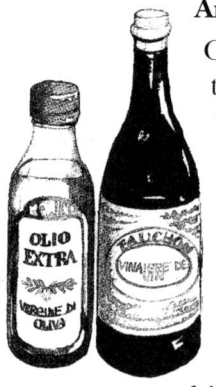

Olive oil has been used for more than 2,000 years as a cleanser and moisturiser for dry skin, and to clean and soothe cuts and scrapes. It is especially useful in eczema. You must use extra virgin oil which is cold pressed olives with no adulteration. This contains more of the healing and soothing substances, such as benzoic acid, which is an antiseptic.

The Romans rubbed themselves with olive oil and then scraped it off with a special tool called a strigil.

....

If you have a mole that is growing, break the branch of a fig tree and rub the sap that oozes out on the mole. It is believed in Iraq that this will stop it growing.

Ahood Al-Rehani

....

Skin care

Natural ingredients

South African women mixed egg yolk with oil and lemon juice and applied it at night if they were going to a wedding or meeting someone. We generally used chicken oil because it is not so thick. Lemon has a bleaching effect, and the oil and yolk nourish the skin. A girl getting married would apply this mixture three times a week.

In addition, they used the South African red earth which they would dig up and make into a ball. It would dry like soft clay and they would break a little off and apply that to their skin for a week at a time – sometimes to the whole body. That was supposed to nourish the body because of the elements in the soil.

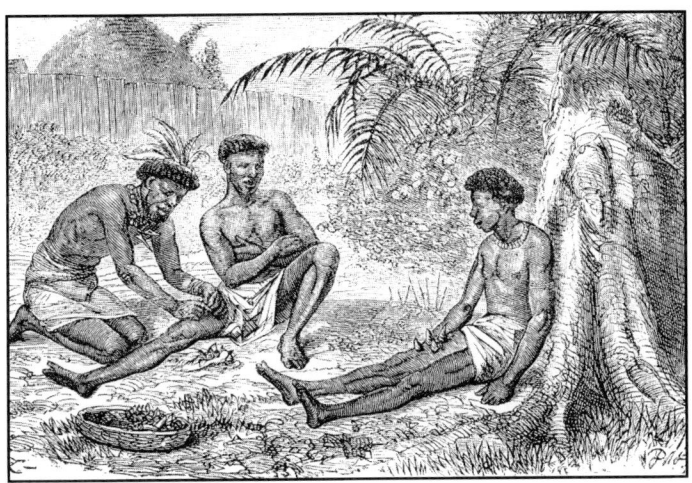

An African medicine man cupping and bleeding two patients   Wellcome Institute Library, London

They also used black sulphur mud which is prevalent in areas of volcanic rock or where there is a hot spring that comes from the earth. Men used this mud as well and it seemed to condition the skin against the sun.

For a natural soap, the South Africans used bulbs. If you cut a hyacinth bulb and rub it, it produces froth; that's what they used to wash their clothes in in olden days.

My mum used to make soap using fat from the pigs, a porridge of cornmeal, maize flour, a colourant, and bitter aloe which also produces froth. But soft soap didn't last.

When the white people came and brought caustic soda, South Africans learned to make soap as we know it. It was a very dangerous operation because caustic soda was lethal and only grown-up ladies would use it. They would cook soap once a year, pour it in shallow dishes and when it was beginning to set, cut it up in desirable sizes. It would last the whole family all year.

Rose Cam

Sores

Chamomile and soap

My Italian mother had a deep sore on her leg. I
remember she cured it with a poultice made from
chamomile leaves. The antiseptic powers of
chamomile were said to be 120 times stronger than
sea water and combined with crushed poppy heads
could be used hot as a fomentation for abscesses
and other swellings.

We also used to rub soap into a sore. Sometimes
we mixed it with sugar and spread it on.

Teresa Mortl

To prevent bed sores (1907)

Beat the white of an egg to a stiff froth, apply to the
tender parts with a piece of cotton-wool or soft rag.
Shake a little starch powder over to prevent sticking.
This is a very simple method and causes no pain.
The egg will keep a long time if put into something
and covered over.

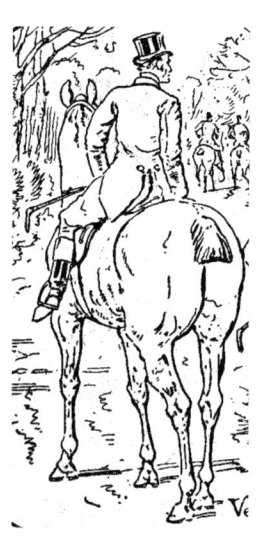

To cure Chaffing occasion'd
by Riding: wash the part
affected with warm Milk
and Water, then anoint it
well with the following
Ointment: one Spoonfull of
Milk, one ditto of Honey,
and one of Brandy, well simmer'd together. Then apply
some white Diacalon
Plaister, spread on white-
brown Paper.
An infallible remedy.

Recommended by Sir John
Knightley, Bart (18th century)

Natural beauty

Natural ingredients, such as fruits, cereals and honey, all of which can be found in the kitchen cupboard or fridge, can be used to make your own beauty preparations cheaply and easily. Remember that they have to be used immediately as they do not contain preservatives and have a very short shelf life.

It is also worth noting that one person's skin may react differently to another's so always do a patch test to ensure you are not allergic to any of the ingredients.

Patch test: Rub a small amount of the ingredients to be used on to an area of the skin which does not show, such as the crook of the arm or behind the ear and leave for up to 12 hours. Allergic reactions include itching, burning redness and swelling. If these occur do not use them.

Pineapple and sunflower scrub

Suitable for normal/oily skin

Mix 1 tbsp. of ground sunflower seeds with 1 tbsp. fresh pineapple juice and 1 tbsp. water. Massage onto the face and neck and leave to dry for 10 mins. Rinse with cool water. (Lemon juice may be substituted for pineapple and has a slight bleaching effect on dull, sallow skin).

Brewers yeast and oatmeal scrub

Suitable for oily blemished skin

Mix 1 tbsp. brewers yeast and 1tbsp. ground oatmeal with enough water to form a paste. Allow the mix to thicken for 1 min. then apply to the face and neck and allow to dry for 15 mins.

Strawberry cleanser

Suitable for all skin types

Mash and strain 4 large ripe strawberries through a fine sieve. Add 2 drops of peppermint essential oil and stir. Massage onto the face and neck avoiding the eye area. Rinse with cool water.

Egg-white face lift

Suitable for mature skin

Beat 1 white of egg with 1 tsp. cornstarch to form stiff peaks. Smooth over the face and neck and leave to dry. As it dries you will feel a tightening effect on the skin. Rinse with cool water.

Peaches and cream mask

Suitable for dry/sensitive skin

Mash a small ripe peach and blend in 1tbsp. thick cream until smooth. Apply to the face and neck and leave for 15mins. Rinse with cool water.

Banana face mask

For normal/dry skin

Peal and mash a small ripe banana. Stir in 1 tbsp. clear honey and 1 tbsp. cream. Apply to the face and neck and leave for 10 mins. Rinse with cool water

Milk bath

Skin softening treatment

Dissolve 4 tbsp. clear honey in 2 pints boiling water and leave to cool. Put 6 tbsp. dried milk powder into a bowl and slowly blend in the honey water. Add to a warm bath and have a relaxing soak.

Anne-Marie Dodson

Stings

Nettles

During my childhood in the 1950s, the only natural cure I remember being told about was the use of dock leaves to ease stings from stinging nettles.

Since we had a sand pit which was part of a disused brickworks behind our house in the Basingstoke Road and this led eventually, over more waste ground, to the River Kennet, the children living in the three terraces opposite the Four Horseshoes Pub often had to use dock leaves, especially in the summer months when vegetation is at its most prolific. Later, I discovered these two plants usually grow near each other.

Daphne Barnes-Phillips

....

Soothe a nettle sting by rubbing with mint, rosemary or dock leaves.

....

Wasp and bee stings

A bluebag for a wasp sting.

A slice of tomato for a bee sting.

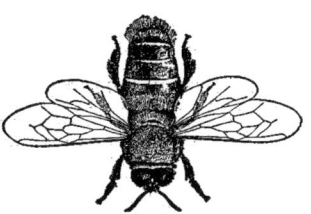

Wet a lump of soda and apply to a wasp or bee sting.

Rub an onion (small ones preferred) on a sting.

'Stung I was'

'Stung I was with a bee on my nose, I presently pluckt out the sting, and layd on honey, so that my face swelled not, thus divine providence reaches to the lowest things. Lett not sin oh Lord that dreadfull sting bee able to poyson mee.' (1644)

The Revd Ralph Josselin, Vicar of Earls Colne, Essex

Jelly-fish and sea urchins

An Australian once told me that urine is the best treatment for jelly fish stings and sea urchin stings. Urine does contain urea which is used in many creams and ointments to moisturise and soften the skin, in conditions like eczema and psoriasis.

Daphne Barnes-Phillips

Warts

Chasing the milkman

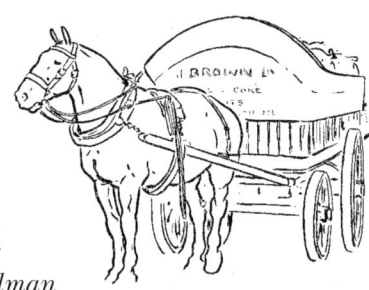

As a child my mother would chase the milk-man's cart and pull a hair from the horse's tail. This would be tied around a wart till it fell off.

Linda Redman

Cut a potato in half, and then rub the wart with it whilst having a conversation with the potato about how you'd like it to remove the wart for you so you can be beautiful again. Once the potato has been well and truly told what its mission in life is, don't throw it away – leave it to rot on a shelf somewhere. By the time the potato has decomposed complete-ly, the wart will have disappeared as well!

Emma Thomas

Rub the wart with radish juice or sloeberry juice twice a day until the wart disappears.

Liquid obtained from the stems of the greater celandine removes warts.

To cure warts, each morning upon waking apply saliva and they will soon disappear.

A lavender revival

Lavender is cultivated for essential oil production across Europe, mostly in France and in Bulgaria, but there are two commercial lavender farms in England, in Hampshire and in Norfolk. A field of gorgeous blue-mauve scented hummocks flowing towards a quintessentially English hedgerow has to be seen to be believed.

The varieties of lavender which are grown commercially in this country are not usually available for gardeners to buy, but they are species of the same hardy *Lavandula angustifolia* which you will probably have in your garden. The oil produced from English lavender has a sweet, honey fragrance, very different from the sharper scent of French lavender.

Some lavender cultivation tips, from the people in Norfolk who know – the plant likes sun and hates wet feet. Don't feed it, don't overwater it, and don't be afraid to cut it back hard after flowering to prevent it from growing gnarled and leggy. It will sprout again from old wood, although many gardening books tell you that it won't. If you're nervous about chopping it back, take a few cuttings first in August or September. Take non-flowering shoots, and plant them in a pot of soil-based compost mixed with sand or vermiculite. You can dip the ends in rooting powder if you have any, but this isn't essential.

Plant lavender around your roses to ward off greenfly, and put a drop of lavender oil on the back of your pet's neck every four to six weeks to keep fleas away!

With the current popularity of aromatherapy and similar gentle, holistic forms of therapy, we are in the middle of a lavender revival, but lavender's cure-all properties have been recognised in Europe for centuries. Perhaps lavender is best known for its sedative, calming properties. After a hard day, a few drops of lavender oil in your bath will relax you and help you unwind. For hard-core insomniacs, put a few drops of oil on your pillow, or burn it in a vaporiser in your bedroom for about 20 minutes before you go to bed – it should give you a peaceful night's sleep.

Lavender oil has other uses. It has a beneficial effect on the immune system and can help to speed recovery from debilitating colds, flu and other illnesses if used in massage or as an inhalation (a few drops floated on a bowl of hot water – cover your head and the bowl with a towel whilst inhaling, to contain the fumes).

It is also one of the very few essential oils which can be applied directly on to the skin with safety. A drop of lavender, rubbed into the temples, will relieve a stress headache and may also reduce the effects of a migraine (make sure that the smell of lavender is acceptable to the sufferer first). It will calm irritated skin and is thought to help cell regeneration. A drop of lavender oil is a useful remedy for minor insect bites and stings, cuts and burns.

Never go on holiday without your lavender oil – adding a few drops to your after-sun lotion will help reduce the effects of sunburn. And rubbing a drop on the sides of your neck, from ears to collarbone, will counteract jet lag. Airline staff are said to swear by this!

Linda Barlow

Thoracic Park

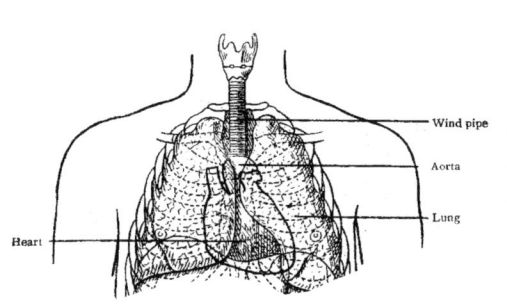

Wind pipe

Aorta

Lung

Heart

'*I*n *Asthma, Chronic Cough,
Influenza, Difficulty of
Breathing, etc., no pen can
describe the wonders that have
been wrought by this deservedly
popular preparation. – Powell's
Balsam of Aniseed.*'

Advertisement c 1909

Chest

Pneumonia

Wrapped in leaves

I was born in Sumatra and lived there until I was 15 years old. In the village where I lived there was a baby who got pneumonia and everyone panicked because it was wartime when there were no doctors about.

A friend of my mother who came from India asked if she could help. She went round the village and collected eggs and she beat them up and made them into omelettes, big round and flat like chapatties.

While they were still warm, the women wrapped them round the baby's arms and legs, tummy and chest, then covered them with warm banana leaves. When banana leaves are warmed they become soft so they don't snap when they are bent, and the women used them like bandages. They gave the baby a spoonful of a mixture made from fresh mint (not too much, just two or three leaves), honey and ground shallots; this was to stop the phlegm.

The baby sweated and slept nicely for three hours and they took off the omelettes and banana leaves and wrapped him in a blanket. The baby was much better the next day.

Dalip Chand

Onions for pneumonia

This remedy was formulated many years ago by one of the best physicians England has ever known, who never lost a patient by the disease and won his renown by simple remedies.

Take six to ten onions according to size and chop finely. Put in a large saucepan over a hot fire, then add the same quantity of rye meal with vinegar enough to form a thick paste. Stir it thoroughly and let it simmer five to ten minutes, then put in a cotton bag large enough to cover the lungs and apply to the chest as hot as the patient can bear. In about 10 minutes, apply another and thus continue by reheating the poultices and in a few hours the patient will be out of danger.

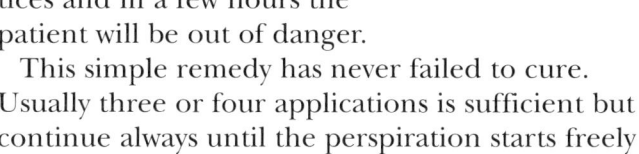

This simple remedy has never failed to cure. Usually three or four applications is sufficient but continue always until the perspiration starts freely from the chest.

Aunt Emily's recipe book

....

An old Mesopotamian formula for treating pneumonia: applications of layers of linseed wrapped in hot compresses, whose heat was renewed by being repeatedly dipped in hot water or hot infusion of fennel.

....

Crisis in the bush

When my twin brother and sister were babies they developed pneumonia.We were living in Australia on the edge of the bush miles away from doctors but my father William McKay Dickson, who had been a medical orderly in the Army in India with the Gordon Highlanders, knew what do.

He wrapped them in brown paper soaked in brandy and walked them up and down all night. The heat was drawn out of the babies and it saved their lives. They are still alive today at the age of 76.

Gladys Bradford

Asthma

Oil and honey
Relief from asthma: mix two ounces of honey with one ounce of castor oil. Take a teaspoon of the mixture each night and morning.

Steaming success
An asthmatic in South Africa would be made to steam in a home-made sauna. The sufferer would sit on a stool over a huge container of boiling water with two or three blankets draped over the head to create a sauna. They got better as they perspired.

Rose Cam

....
Encourage an asthmatic child to blow soap bubbles. Blowing and taking deep breaths helps to extend the chest cavity.
....

Bronchitis

Moravian wise women
Moravian woods and meadows conceal many special treasures which have been used for centuries to cure a great variety of human and animal ailments.

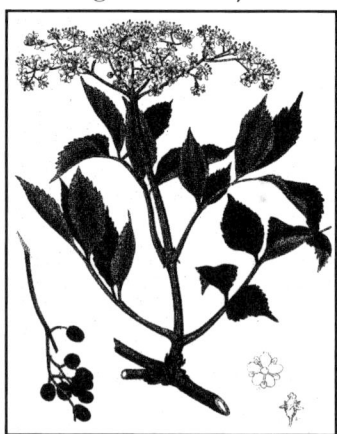

Elder flowers help bronchitis

Legend has it that women of mystery and wonderful knowledge used to live in their dwellings far from other people. Some called them witches, others said they were women of great wisdom. Not only did they cure many ills, but they also shared their knowledge with ordinary folks.

Children suffering from bronchitis would be given a rather bitter infusion made from European elder flowers. It did taste foul but it stopped persistent coughing. The only problem was to catch the child and make him drink their healing potion.

Little patients affected by whooping cough were bathed in extract from pine needles. This calmed the cough and their mothers could sleep peacefully but not the children! They turned into silent walking ghosts in their sleep. Their fever was gone at daybreak and they looked quite human again.

Moy Trchalik

....

We used brown paper and goose grease for our chests – if you had a goose!

Cyril Shuffle, 91

....

Whooping cough

Tar fumes

Children with whooping cough or some other chest trouble would be taken to breath tar fumes.

Marsh Mallow

The Romans are supposed to have introduced marsh mallow plants to Britain.

Boiled in wine or milk, marsh mallow was a popular remedy for whooping cough, bronchitis and other diseases of the chest, frequently given in the form of a syrup.

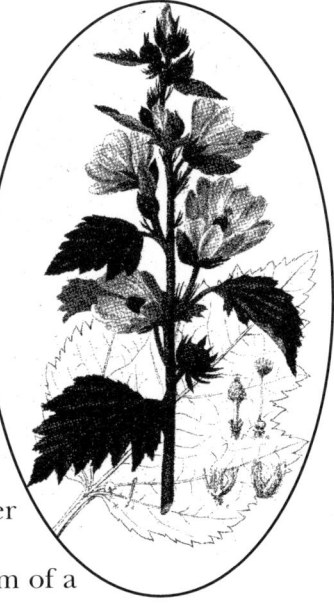

Marsh mallow

Nonna

Adalgisa Polli 'Nonna Dalgisa', my paternal grandmother, was born in 1902, in the South Tyrol which was then part of the Austro-Hungarian empire. In 1918 it was claimed by Italy but Nonna remained fiercely Austrian all her life and did not like Italians.

Life was very hard particularly after her husband died and she struggled to raise three small children in Italy. When illness struck she could not afford a doctor so she relied on the knowledge that she had learned from her mother and treated her family with herbs and home-made lotions and tinctures.

She passed this on to us when she came to live with my parents in Reading in 1959.

Although she couldn't cook, burning everything she touched apart from strudel and potato gnocchi, she did make sure that we ate a varied diet. It was probably higher in fat than recommended today but as children we were very active and soon burned it off. We always had fresh vegetables and fruit after every meal and what little meat we had was of the best quality. Her favourite recipes for a convalescent were beef broth and chicken soup.

South Tyroleans are obsessed with regularity. If I did not go every day I was given a tea made from senna pods or given syrup of figs with explosive results. Even today my father still swears by castor oil and Epsom salts.

Modern medicine now frowns upon regular use of laxatives, saying that it can lead to severe constipation which can in turn lead to haemorrhoids. In my grandmother's day bad haemorrhoids were cauterised with a red hot poker. My grandmother was convinced that to avoid piles you had to be regular. If she discovered that I had not been for more than two days she resorted to soap suppositories – quite simply pieces of soap chopped off a large bar and softened and shaped, if I was lucky!

I was a healthy child, albeit slight, but my grandmother was convinced that I was frail and tried her best to build me up. For breakfast I was given zabaglione, a raw egg yolk beaten into a small glass of marsala. We were all given this when recovering from any illness. My mother would give me a small glass before exams. It probably did nothing for my health but it certainly calmed me down.

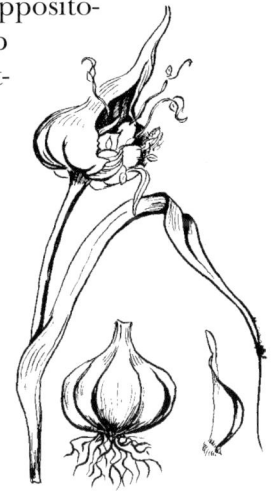

Garlic

When Nonna wasn't dosing us with laxatives she was brewing up valerian tea. Valerian was widely used on the continent as mild sedative and you can now buy it in tablet form. The part used was the root which is washed, peeled and simmered with boiling water to produce the foulest herbal drink in existence. It works but it stinks the house out.

Whenever I had flu as a teenager, Nonna used to lace hot milk with schnapps, smear my chest and back with Vick and then order me to bed with as many blankets and hot-water bottles as I could stand, the idea being to sweat out the disease. She sometimes made her own infusions of herbs in grappa. The one I remember most vividly because of its bitter taste was rue – good for getting rid of worms and for inducing a sweat. Other ingredients would be juniper berries and the buds of a particular conifer, although I only saw them being picked in Italy.

It seems that most of the remedies she concocted were incredibly bitter although an alcoholic drink made from lemon verbena and used for digestive problems was very pleasant. I think Nonna just drank it because she liked it.

Nonna would dip a bandage in fresh urine and then used it to treat sprained wrists and ankles. For some reason it had to be donated by the youngest child in the house and the duty used to fall on my youngest sister who would always balk at the request. If there was no urine she used egg white. Either way the bandage would start to contract as it dried. It was very strange, but did seem to work. Perhaps the irritation it caused was greater than the pain from the injury.

I remember getting threadworm when I was six. Nonna's cure was to send us to bed with necklaces of peeled garlic and to use a peeled clove as a suppository. Needless to say I soon learned to wash my hands thoroughly before eating. She also used to make a bitter tasting tea which I now know to be rue. It grows well in this country but be careful when handling it as it can cause an allergic reaction.

No matter what the season we always rounded off a meal with a serving of salad greens, fresh from the garden. We ate rugola, dandelion leaves, endive, chicory and red oak leaf salad long before they became trendy. Nonna said that it aided digestion and helped you sleep. I have since discovered that wild lettuce has narcotic properties and the milky juice that exudes from a cut in its stem was once dried and used as a sedative.

So I grew up taking home cures for granted. I thought everyone drank chamomile tea to help them sleep or had bottles of herbal tinctures macerating in their airing cupboards.

Linda Maestranzi

Rue

Hiccoughs

Some simple cures

Tickle your nose with a feather to induce a sneeze.

Drink in one gulp a large glass of water in which there is an eggspoon.

Take a teaspoon of fresh lemon juice.

Drink the juice of half an orange.

Take teaspoonful doses of onion juice.

Chew a leaf of fresh tarragon or mint.

Hold your breath and count to 20 slowly.

Swallow a small piece of ice.

Drink some gripe water.

Chew caraway seeds

Mint

Breathe in and out of a paper bag 20 times.

Drink a glass of water from the opposite side of the glass. Stretch your arms above your head while someone gives you a glass of water.

Apply a hot-water bottle to the pit of the stomach.

Suck a lump of sugar or swallow one teaspoon of vinegar.

Heart

A clove of garlic a day

My mother swallows a clove of fresh garlic every day as she did in Iraq. It's good for the heart.

Ahood Al-Rehani

Summer Love Potion

Red carnations are a powerful symbol of love, and borage has an age-old reputation for giving the heart courage and gladdening the senses. John Evelyn, writing in the 17th century, said: "Sprigs of Borage are of known virtue to revive the hypochondriac and cheer the hard student."

Take: the petals of nine dark red carnations, three borage leaves and as many flowers, a bottle of champagne or sparkling wine. Open the champagne. Insert the leaves and flowers. Leave to infuse for several hours in a fridge.

To stop the wine from going flat, suspend a silver spoon in the neck of the bottle. Strain into glasses.

Lungs

Lungwort, a member of the borage family, used to be found in almost every garden under the name of Jerusalem Cowslip. It was reputed to have medicinal qualities in diseases of the lungs but Sir J E Smith, founder of the Linnaean Society, said that "every part of the plant is mucilaginous, but its reputation for coughs arose not from this circumstance, but from the speckled appearance of the leaves resembling lungs!" An infusion of one teaspoonful of the dried herb to a cup of boiling water can be taken for subduing inflammation, and pulmonary complaints.

Lungwort

Brother Cadfael's Herbs

Although Brother Cadfael, the twelfth century monk of Shrewsbury Abbey, was the ficitional creation of Ellis Peters in a series of mystery and detective novels, the herbs he grew are known and still used today.

In his famous herb garden in the Abbey, he nurtured more than fifty herbs and plants from which he made salves and lotions for the monks and any of the citizens of Shrewsbury who came to ask for his help.

Understandably, a great many of the requests he had were for syrups to soothe the coughs and colds frequent throughout the winter months. Monastic life was hard and had few comforts. Buildings were mostly unheated and the monks, particularly the older brothers, suffered in the cold weather.

Brother Cadfael made a syrup of rosemary and rue, or coltsfoot, for coughs; used bay and borage in mulled wine for bad chests. He also used goosegrease and mustard as a poultice for chesty coughs. Almond oil was used for chapped hands, a very common problem, and wintergreen for a soothing lotion, perhaps for chilblains.

Powdered hyssop root was another herb used for chest troubles and jaundice, but this had to be used with great care, as a large dose could kill. It was also used, in those days, along with the iris known as fleur de luce, to procure abortions. Of course, Cadfael would never have used the plants for this purpose, though he did know their uses.

Saxifrage

Cadfael's second most commonly requested remedy was soothing oils to ease the aches and pains of the older monks. One can imagine that "the rheumatics" were commonplace among all but the youngest brothers! For this he used houseleek as an ingredient in an oil for rubbing into the skin to ease aching joints. His preferred treatment was with monkshood, mixed with oil, which could be massaged deep into aching joints to relieve the pain. This was, however, an extremely poisonous plant, which had to be handled with great care, as only a very small amount could prove fatal if ingested.

Another common medical problem Brother Cadfael was called upon to treat was rheum in the eyes, for which he used saxifrage, or linseed oil from flax, and horehound, which could also be used for coughs and colds. He concocted a soothing syrup from orpine, *Sedum telephium,* for raging quinsy, used mulberry leaves as a paste for burns, made a soothing ointment from mandrake root, and used lady's mantle for burns and bed sores.

Occasionally, Cadfael had to treat less common problems. He used hound's tongue in a lotion to counteract a dog's bite (probably a good deal more serious in the 12th century than now) and lavender for disorders of the head or spirit, which could have meant emotional distress. A mixture of mint and sorrel vinegar could be sniffed as a restorative after dizziness and fainting.

He used trefoil (a clover) to strengthen the heart after a seizure, though he doesn't seem

Clover

to have used foxglove (digitalis). His herbal skills were practised on many of the citizens of the town, and their children. He made a concoction of dill and fennel which relieved wind in a baby's stomach. Does dill water still stir the memory today?

The Brother Cadfael books span the period 1137–1144, when the civil war between King Stephen and the Empress Maud was at its height. He therefore needed many salves to dress and cleanse wounds, and to treat ulcerated wounds, which were a common occurrence with neglect or old injuries.

Dill

He used sanicle for cleansing wounds; marsh mallow, St John's wort, moneywort and white deadnettle for dressing wounds. Comfrey was also used, and was particularly effective against gout.

As well as herbs for culinary purposes to improve the flavour of the Abbot's dinners, Cadfael grew several plants solely for their perfume, such as violets, rue, lily of the valley, jasmine and clover. These were used to perfume the oils used in the altar lamps and Abbey candles, though Cadfael was also known to give perfumed oils unofficially to certain favoured ladies of his acquaintance.

Betty O'Rourke

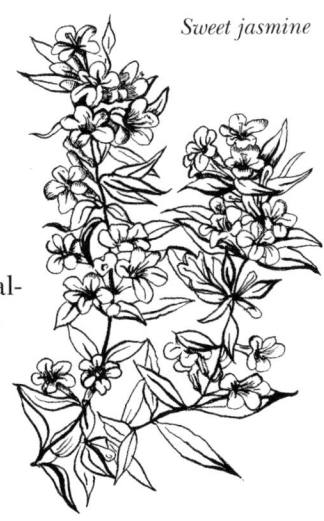

Sweet jasmine

■ The Brother Cadfael books by Ellis Peters are published by Hodder Headline

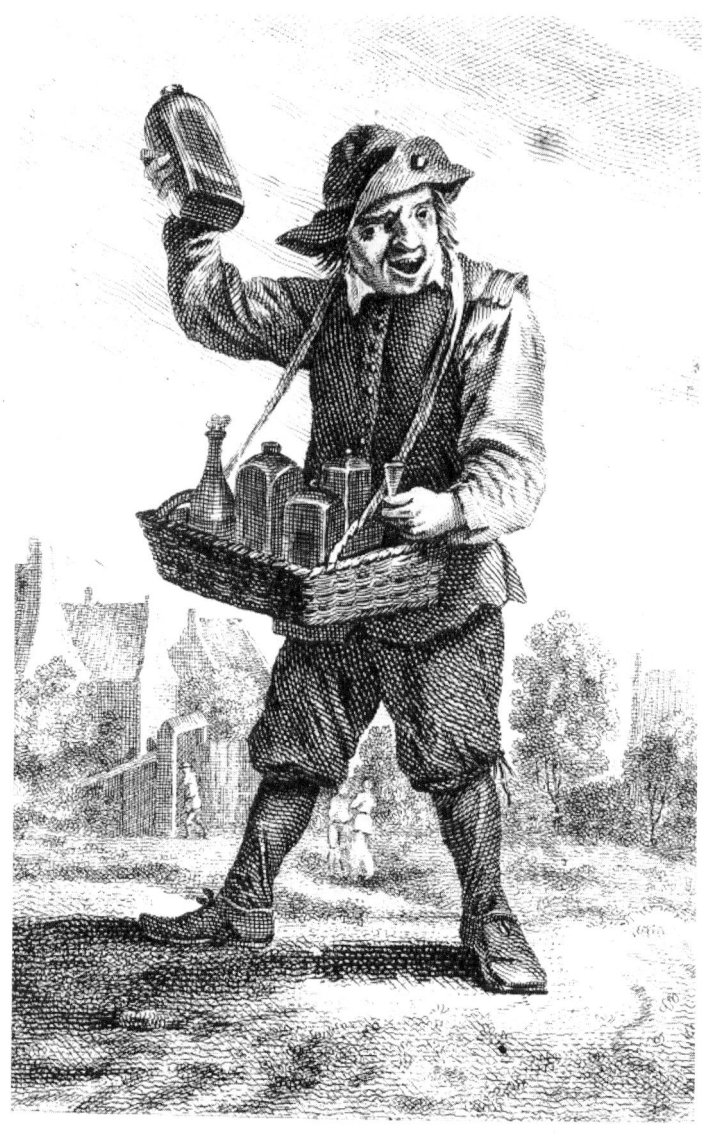

*An itinerant seller of medicines – an etching by T Kitchen
(18th century) after David Teniers (1582-1649)*

Wellcome Institute Library, London

*W*ind and *W*ater

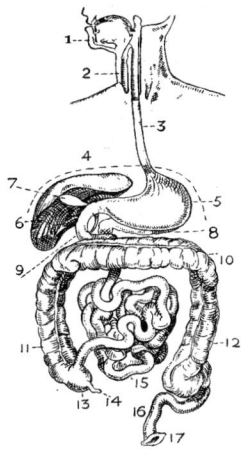

'*W*helpton's Vegetable
Purifying Pills *arouse*
the stomach to action, promote
the flow of gastric juice, and give
tone to the whole system.'

Advertisement c 1912

Stomach

Digestion and indigestion

Cleansing the body

In South Africa we used castor oil in addition to Epsom salts to cleanse the body because we ate a lot of meat. As soon as we had eaten meat, my grandmother used an enema.

We had amasi every day, sour milk like yogurt which we made ourselves. We believed it had an effect on the heart and helped it to be healthy. We grew our own sugar beans and kidney beans and we would pick wild beans, tiny but so sweet, and chew them in autumn and winter when they had dried in their pods.

Rose Cam

....

Nutritionists have now confirmed what my Italian mother always claimed – that olive oil is good for you. It contain amino acids that are very similar to those found in human breast milk and so is ideal for young children or anyone with poor digestion. I added a teaspoon to all the savoury purées that I served up to my babies – I even added it to any prepared foods I used. My mother said that it was better drizzled over and taken raw than being added while the food is being cooked.

Linda Maestranzi

....

Cures for indigestion

One teaspoonful of essence of peppermint, rhubarb powder and bicarbonate of soda, one pint of boiling water added slowly. One tablespoonful after meals for indigestion.

If I ever get indigestion, I eat liquorice.

Teresa Mortl

Pain about the belly

This is a very common complaint among sailors, who will come aft complaining of wind on the stomach and pain about the belly after meals. It may be due to the monotony of shipboard food continued for any length of time, and is also frequently caused by bad teeth.

Give 20 grains of bicarbonate of potash and 10 drops of essence of peppermint in a wineglassful of water after each meal.

The Ship Captain's Medical Guide (1912)

After a heavy meal, drink an infusion of sage – a few leaves in a cup of boiling water, or try an infusion of a pinch of aniseed in a cup of boiling water. An infusion of a pinch of aniseed and one of cumin in a cup of boiling milk will relieve painful flatulence, so will stewed parsley or stewed mint. Eating charcoal – toast burnt black for instance – will also help.

Mint

Freed of that great oppression

'This night about one of the clock I fell ill of a surfeit occasioned by drinking water after venison. I was great oppressed in my stomach and next day Mr Saunders the Astrologian sent me a piece of Briony root to hold in my hand and within a quarter of an hour my stomach was freed of that great oppression.'

Elias Ashmole (1617-92), antiquarian

Potato juice

For indigestion, drink the juice of a grated potato that has been allowed to stand for an hour or so.

Ala Zolkiewka from Poland

Rich food, light food

During the winter in Pakistan, we ate all kinds of rich food, chicken and meat to keep warm and every year when spring came we would be given a laxative to clean the stomach. In the summer, when it was so hot, we ate much lighter food. We'd have vegetables, dahl, and cool yogurt drinks.

In the winter, my father made a sort of pudding of carrots, nuts, preserved fruit and egg yolks. It kept for weeks and we'd help ourselves to it freely.

We would also eat preserved fruit wrapped in a piece of gold or silver, beaten so thin that it would just crumble as you ate it. That was meant to give you strength.

Akhtar Aziz

Learning from the birds

In Persia [Iran] it was believed that medical knowledge was a direct revelation from God or observations of God's world. The clyster, or enema syringe, was introduced after a pelican was observed in great distress after having over-indulged from a shoal of small fishes. The pelican filled his long beak with water and proceeded to administer to himself a high enema relieving the pain from its stomach. The observer successfully used this method on patients suffering from gastric problems.

Upset stomach

You need a dried lime – you can get it from Indian shops. Crush it and make a drink with hot water. Leave it to simmer just like tea and drink it with sugar. It settles the stomach miraculously if you are feeling queasy.

Ahood Al-Rehani

'To Indigestion Wind in the Stomack'

A pint of brandy, an ounce of sliced rhubarb, half an ounce of powdered jesuits bark, half an ounce of lesser cardamom powder, a quarter ounce of Seville orange peel, infused together for two days, then filtered through paper and another half pint of brandy added. This to be left another week, then filtered. The dose is a dessertspoonful after dinner.

The Benyon family of Englefield (18th and 19th century)

'Yesterday having wetted my feet by walking out in the dew and having eaten a small piece of new cheese, I have been today tortured with flatulent spasms. By taking two doses of hiera picra [a purgative drug composed of aloes and canella bark] the pains in my stomach abated. Thanks to the great God for his mercy towards me.'

Aloe

Timothy Burrell (1643-1717)

Good for the blood

Every spring in Switzerland my grandmother would make a concoction of herbs to clean the blood – I know it contained walnut leaves.

Dandelion is also good for this. You can eat the young leaves like a salad. A tisane made from chamomile flowers is good for upset stomachs but don't add sugar.

Joan Head

A Recpt for the Stomach when stuff'd with Phlegm: Ipecacuanha and Rhubarb of each 5 grains, mix'd in any Liquid; to be taken in the Morning fasting.

Dr Jenner of Berkeley (of vaccination fame)

For a Bilious complaint

Take a new laid egg, mash the whole of it well and take it an hour before breakfast. It has been known to make a perfect cure by taking it six or eight weeks.

From Mary Loder's recipe book (18th century).

Bitter sweet

Italians, like many Europeans, swear by bitters – pungent alcoholic herbal infusions that they believe aid digestion, improve lost appetites and help upset stomachs, especially when accompanied by hangovers. Many of these bitters were first produced by monastic orders.

The more commercial ones are milder in flavour and not as medicinal but are still made from herbs and spices steeped in alcohol and then sweetened. I always have a bottle of Fernet Branca which I mix with warm water and a spoon of sugar when I have eaten too much or feel sick. Campari, which is drunk before meals to stimulate the appetite, and Pimms are even milder versions.

I also mix a few drops of Angostura Bitters with tonic water when I have overindulged. This is not alcoholic and helps morning sickness.

Linda Maestranzi

Kidneys

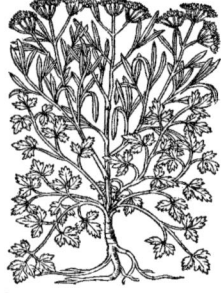
Parsley

Moravian mixture

Inflammatory diseases of the urinary tract and the kidneys could be helped by drinking an extract from birch leaves, mint leaves and parsley. This mixture which we use in Moravia is fast working and effective.

Moy Trchalik

God be thanked

'A great fit of the stone in my left kydney; all day I could do but three or four drops of water but I drunk a draught of whit wyne and salet oyle and after that crab's eyes in powder with the bone in the carps head and abowt four of the clok I did eat tosted cake buttered and with sugar and nutmeg on it and drunk two great draughts of ale with it and I voyded within an howr much water and a stone as big as an Alexander stone. God be thanked.'

Dr John Dee (1527-1604), mathematician and alchemist

Spinach and sea kale

Mother Jame, a wise-woman living in Oxfordshire in the 19th century, used to make a concoction from grasses, spinach and dandelion (sometimes with a small quantity of sea kale) to combat kidney disorders.

Tony Barham

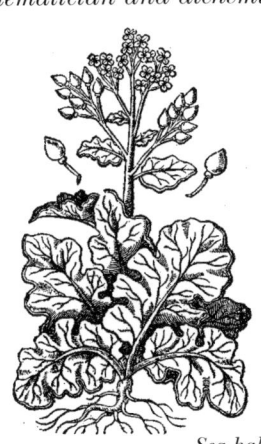
Sea kale

17th century New England remedy

Recipe to prevent or cure a stone in the kidneys or bladder: take wild carrot seeds and boil them in ale, then drink a dose three times every night.

'The Bishop assured mee that faire spring water in the morning receaved into your mouth and there kept untill itt bee lukewarme and then swallowed is an excellent medicine to cure the cholick and stone and that hee himself had been hereby cured.'

Sir William Brereton, a Parliamentarian during the Civil War who kept a diary in 1634 and 1635

Constipation

Feeling seedy?

For constipation people from Pakistan use Sat-Isabqol, a natural vegetable product derived from Isabqol seeds by milling, or onion seeds, mixed with water or orange juice.

Akhtar Aziz

Prune juice is an ancient remedy for constipation and fig juice for sickness of the stomach and bowels.

For this relief ...

Many continentals are not as squeamish as Britons when it comes to suppositories which they regard as more effective than tablets, since the medication is absorbed more quickly into the bloodstream.

When my son was immobilised in a cast from toe to chest for a broken leg he became constipated. Nothing that the doctors gave us worked so we resorted to traditional medicine. Three times each day he had a tablespoon of boiled sieved prunes. Then our neighbour advised me to make a suppository from softened soap and the pounded leaves of a type of marsh mallow. It was unpleasant but it took effect within two days.

Fig

Linda Maestranzi

Patients may take a glass of hot water with great benefit every morning before breakfast. Constipated people are generally found to drink very little water

'Get Back to Nature and Live' C W Aloysius Browne

Diarrhoea

A little rice

Rice carefully boiled in water taken with a little salt as the only food for 48 hours, and the boiled rice water cold as the only drink often cuts short an attack especially when the diarrhoea is due to fruit or climatic influence. Drink plenty of rice water when thirsty. This is a common remedy in Italy.

The R.E.P. Book (1903)

Let the patient take all his food and drink cold while the relaxed condition of the bowels continues. No meat, hot tea, coffee or cocoa should be taken. Cold arrowroot tea made with milk is excellent.

'Get Back to Nature and Live' C W Aloysius Browne

Drink lemon juice and sweet, strong black coffee.

....

Eat nothing for 24 hours then only plain boiled rice until symptoms abate. For a day or two eat only plain food. An Indian hint is to eat a thin gruel made from oats or chapatties or dry toast.

....

Secret weapon

During the Second World War, soldiers from New Zealand took koromiko plants with them to the Middle East as a remedy for dysentery.

There is an enormous number of varieties of the koromiko (Hebe species), which is a smallish bush with white or lilac flowers shaped like bottle brushes. The young leaves of the koromiko, if eaten raw, cure diarrhoea and the young shoots, when chewed, relieve stomach pains. The cooked root of the New Zealand bracken fern also alleviates diarrhoea and calms an upset stomach.

Something to glory in

I was a healthy child growing up in Jamaica and used to bathe a lot in the sea. If we had upset stomach, we would have a drink of ginger and cerasee, which grows like a vine, infused in boiling water. That opened your bowels. You've got to clear your bowels every day or you wonder what's wrong.

When I was small my mother made a drink of strong salts, a lime or two and a pinch of sugar, put it in a bottle and shook it well and every morning we would have a wine glass full. That cleared your insides and took care of coughs and colds and pimples and bumps. If my stomach hurt or I hadn't opened my bowels, my mother would look into my eyes and say, "You have worms". Then I would have a medicine made of a little weed and after two or three doses I would pass the worms.

If you couldn't sleep you would put a leaf or two of soursop under your pillow or tie it on your head and you'd sleep. You can get soursop over here now. You can peel it like an orange and eat it, or it makes a nice drink. You could boil up bitterwood and make a medicine from it. There was a herb or plant for everything.

In 1914 there was an epidemic of chickenpox where we lived and the doctors closed their surgeries and came down into the country to pick herbs and plants

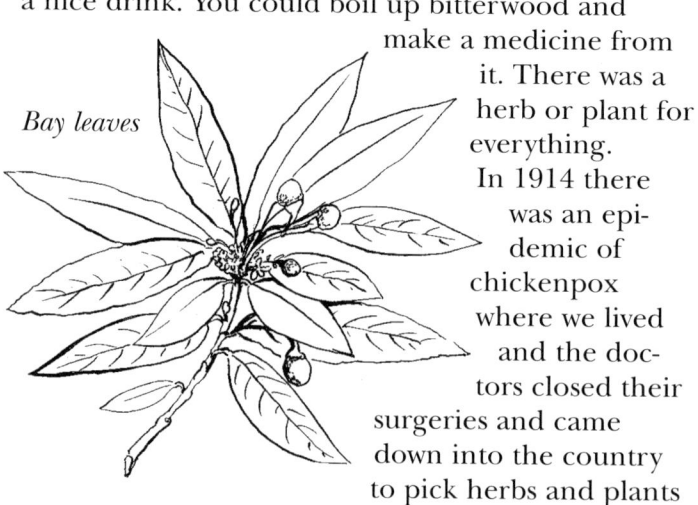

Bay leaves

to make medicines to cure the people.

I am 90 now. Why have I lived so long? The secret is that I know myself. As I grow older the Lord tells me what to do. He watches over me and tells me when I am not up to par. The first thing to do is to find what is the cause of your trouble.

This morning I woke up and my eyes were not feeling so wonderful. It's because I don't take as much exercise as I used to do, I sit inside and watch *Neighbours*. So I go out and walk about in the fresh air and that refreshes my eyes. I wasn't feeling so well the other day and the voice told me, "You must rest at midday". I wasn't thinking of resting, I had so many things to do, but I have learned to let things go.

If it is time to have a drink, your body tells you and you better do it. If I am fast asleep and I wake up at 3.30 am then I will have a cup of tea.

I eat carefully: vegetables, fish is my delight, a little meat, chiefly chicken, cheese and fruit, and milk. I like things nice and delicate and mostly fresh.

I have a plant growing on my windowsill called the Leaf of Life and I put that on my eyes or my head if they hurt. You can rub it, squeeze it and drink it. It's a cure for everything.

I drink Aloe Vera and that's cooling and refreshing. My hair is getting thin now and I rub my head if it's hot with bay rum, which is rum with a bay leaf in it. That cools my brain!

Life's not all sunshine, it would not be Christianity if it was. You have to have something to glory in, someone to be grateful to. People aren't taught to say thank-you any more.

My mother taught me:
Hearts like doors are ope with ease,
With very, very little keys
"I thank you, sir" and "If you please".

'Mother' Agatha Walker

Invalid diet

A good cook is half a doctor - Culpepper

Beef tea

Scrape or cut half a pound of meat as small as possible. Put it into an earthenware basin. Pour over it half a pint of cold water, and cover it with paper bound tightly round the edges. Place in the hollow of a slow oven for an hour, add salt, and strain off.

Gruel

Sprinkle into one quart of boiling water three tablespoonfuls of oatmeal and a pinch of salt. Simmer slowly for an hour, then strain.

Barley water

Wash a handful of pearl barley in cold water, then simmer it in three pints of water for an hour, and flavour with a little lime-juice and sugar.

Imperial drink

Dissolve half an ounce of Cream of Tartar in one quart of boiling water, and flavour with lime-juice and sugar. This is a very cooling drink in fevers.

Toast water

A crust of bread must be toasted till it is almost black, then cold water is poured on it and the whole allowed to stand.

The Ship Captain's Medical Guide (1912)

Eggs for an invalid

For preparing eggs for an invalid, try this method. Beat the yolk and white separately until extremely light, add a pinch of salt, pour into a china cup, which set in a saucepan of hot water, stirring constantly till scalded, but not cooked. When this is done the cup is almost filled with creamy custard. Set in the oven a moment and serve at once.

French sick dishes

Recipe collections of the late middle ages often contained dishes suitable for the sick. One book of 1420 offered 16 recipes for sick dishes. The first one is called a restorative in which one or two capons are cooked with pearls, pieces of gold and a broad selection of gemstones.

....

'Was taken with a violent ague – drank hot punch and Madeira negus [wine and hot water, sweetened, and flavoured with lemon and spice] – found myself heavy with that – slept well rest of night; drank much milk and water, wonderfully refreshing – which sat pleasingly on my stomach.'

'Awoke ce matin with a violent pain... took warm water, honey, rum, turlington, then a mug of warm water and souring then wood strawberry brandy. However eat nothing but a little broth to dinner and at picquet broad glass of gin punch and turlington. Afterwards mug small beer and sugar – to bed soon after ten.'

John Baker (1712-1777)

....

Healthy food and tonics

Rations for good health

(post-Second World War hints)

Ingredients:
half a pint of milk, 1oz cheese, 1oz bacon, 1 egg, 6 slices of brown and white bread, 1 orange, 1 level tablespoon of cocoa (or 1oz of chocolate).

Collect all ingredients on a tray daily, and eat your way through them. Add liver once a week and fat fish (herrings, mackerel, sardines) once a week. This is what your body needs. Add what you like though keep off too many cakes, sweets and biscuits and too much fat, sugar and meat. Result: good health.

Rosemary remedy

Rosemary has long been held to stimulate the brain – ancient Greek scholars wore garlands of rosemary to help them think clearly. This remedy is meant to restore concentration and mental energy and will combat tension, stress and tiredness.

Take 25g of freshly picked rosemary, a sealable jar or bottle, rosemary oil, one tablespoon of unperfumed skin lotion

Boil one litre of water. Add the fresh rosemary (flowers or sprigs – it all works). Leave for ten minutes to infuse. Strain into the jar or bottle. Drink three cups a day, sweeten with honey if desired.

To stimulate your senses and keep you alert, blend two drops of rosemary oil with the skin lotion and rub on to the temples.

A pick-me-up

Take four new-laid eggs, squeeze the juice of four lemons on them, cover and leave three or four days till the shells are soft, then beat up all together and strain through muslin. Add a quarter pint of new milk, beating well, then half a pint of rum. Still beating, add another quarter pint of milk. Bottle and keep corked. Shake the bottle before taking a wine glass twice a day.

Aunt Emily's recipes

Recipe for Centerbe liqueur (a cure-all)

Three each of bay leaves, juniper berries, chamomile flowers, cloves, coffee-beans, one orange leaf, basil, lemon balm, mint, rosemary, sage, lime, thyme (and any other fresh herbs you happen to have around), one stick of cinnamon, four pieces of saffron, 500 ml Polish vodka, or pure alcohol if you can get it, 350g sugar.

Mix all ingredients except sugar in a large jar, shake and leave to infuse in a warm place for one month. Filter into a large bottle. Boil 500 ml of water with the sugar until it becomes syrupy. When cool add to bottle. Cork and store for at least three months before using.

Thyme

Pick-me-ups

Infuse lemon verbena in boiling water.

Marguerite Hudson, Australia

Take the juice of half a lemon, a lump or two of sugar, water and a few drops of essence of ginger; or a tablespoon or two of ginger syrup to a gill of water, favoured with lime- or lemon-juice. (1907)

....

To Create a Stomake [sic] or for one in a wasting Condishon 6 live vipers or 8 dried ones, 2 ounces each of flower of rosemary and lavender and one ounce of bruised winter's bark in 3 quarts of strong white wine for 3-4 months, then strained. A glass twice a day, before dinner and supper.

18th century

....

Dry'd Orange Peel and Rosemary, good for nervous complaints, taken for breakfast about half a pint.

Dr Ash

Shenachrum and Samson

Writing in 1888 Sir Arthur Quiller-Couch tells of
two restorative drinks from the Fowey area of
Cornwall used for people suffering from shock, particularly for those near to drowning. Shenachrum
consisted of beer, rum, sugar and lemon all heated
together, and Samson was brandy, cider and sugar.

Samson can be made with his hair on or not.
Since Samson was stronger before his hair was cut,
Samson with hair has a double quantity of brandy.

Tony Barham

Fighting over lime blossoms

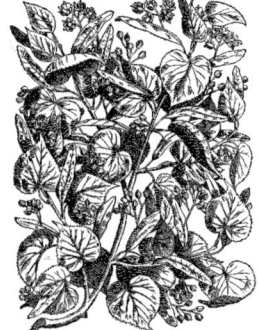

'Dr Chandler tells that in the south
of France an infusion of the blos-
soms of the lime tree, *Tilia*, is in
much esteem as a remedy for
coughs, hoarseness, fevers, etc., and
that at Nismes, he saw an avenue of
limes that was quite ravaged and
torn in pieces by people greedily
gathering the bloom, which they
dried and kept for these purposes.

Lime tree   'Upon the strength of this information
we made some tea of limeblossoms, and found it a
very soft, well-flavoured, pleasant, saccharine julep,
in taste much resembling the juice of liquorice.'

The Rev Gilbert White of Selborne (1720-1793)

If you are stressed, depressed, anxious, and unable
to sleep, eat a bowl of porridge. Oats not only lower
blood cholesterol levels, but they are also good for
the nervous system. Try putting a cupful of oats into
a muslin bag or a pair of tights and tie it onto the
taps before running a bath. The warm water will
relax you, and the oats calm sensitive or itchy skin.

Emma Thomas

Jewish Penicillin

That's what they call chicken soup. Just the smell of a well-made chicken broth is enough to lift your spirits – good health soon follows.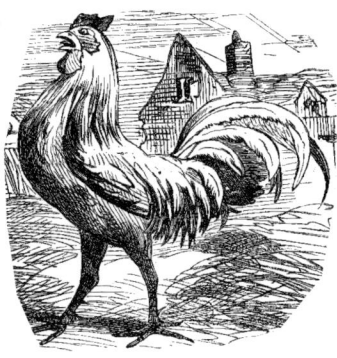

The recipes vary according to the country of origin but the basic ingredients are a good meaty chicken (not too young but not so old that it is stringy), two onions, two to three stalks of celery and carrots, parsley and dill. Bring to boil and simmer for two to three hours until the chicken is tender. Remove it and strain.

Linda Maestranzi

Herbal teas are popular in Portugal and can help many ailments. We drink infusions of basil, which has a calming effect on the nervous system and also aids digestion, hypericum or St John's wort for intestinal problems, and coriander and mint which both improve digestion. Thyme is good for sore throats and coughs (and so are onion skins). Nettles cleanse the blood and parsley helps the circulation and purifies bad breath. Pes de cerjos – the skin of cherries – is good for urinary infections and we drink lemon and honey for constipation and influenza.

Isabel Sottomajor

Calves' foot jelly and sympathy

My father worked as a chauffeur and steward in private service for a family living in Whitchurch. We had a cottage on the estate and if we were ill, they came from the big house with bowls of soup and calves' foot jelly.

Cyril Shuffle, aged 91

Sage the Saviour

Sage or *Salvia officinalis* is native to the
Mediterranean region but has been cultivated
for culinary and medicinal purposes for many
centuries in England, France and Germany.
Cultivated sage comes in many forms but for medicinal purposes the red sage *Salvia officinalis*
'Purpurascens' and the broad-leaved white (or
green sage) have been proved to be the best.

Sage was so highly regarded that it was spoken of
as Salvia salvatrix (sage the saviour). A saying, probably Arabian, but quoted in Spanish universities in
the Middle Ages, "Cur moriatur homo cui salvia cre-
sit in horto?" (Why should a man die whilst sage
grows in his garden?), has an English equivalent:
"He that would live for aye must eat sage in May."

It was believed to have mystical properties too and
Samuel Pepys recorded how graves in the
Southampton area were sown with sage since the
plant was thought to mitigate grief.

Powerful herb

This versatile herb has an enormous range of
medicinal uses but be warned: one of its components is camphor so although the plant is safe the
volatile oil should be treated with great caution.

Sage acts as a powerful tonic. Components of the
leaves and flowers increase the circulation of the
blood and help the nervous system. In 1995 sage oil
was found to inhibit the enzyme acetylcholin-
esterase, thought to contribute to the memory loss
characteristic of Alzheimer's disease.

As sage is a diuretic, an antispasmodic and a
restorative it can be used to treat sluggish kidneys,
oedema, gout, rheumatism and migraine.

It reduces fever in infectious illnesses, helps to
maintain the right hormonal balance and is helpful

in cases of diabetes. A decoction will rapidly bring the blood sugar back to normal.

There are compounds in sage which appear to have an inhibiting effect on the organisms which cause septicaemia, cholera and dysentry.

Sage heals wounds, speeds up the formation of a scab and is a powerful antiseptic used externally. As a gargle it is recommended for gingivitis, inflammation of the throat and palate, thrush, tonsillitis in children, dental caries and abscesses.

Used as a lotion or compress or in a bath it helps wounds, ulcers, boils, chilblains, sprains and pulled muscles.

A lotion for ulcers

A strong infusion without lemon or sugar helps to heal raw abrasions of the skin and can be used as a lotion for ulcers. Flowers and leaves of sage can be made into a strong decoction. Add five tablespoons of the sage to one litre of cold water, cover and bring slowly to the boil. Boil for ten minutes, infuse for a further ten minutes before straining. This is good for mouth ulcers and a sore throat.

As a steam bath, sage has an astringent effect on the skin and at the same time eases severe head colds and coughs, thanks to its disinfectant, antiviral and expectorant properties.

To help the respiratory tract take one handful of whole or shredded sage leaves, one handful of peppermint leaves, one handful of whole lime flowers, and a small handful of chamomile flowers. Basil, elderflowers and lavender can also be added.

Pour boiling water over the mixture and inhale in the usual manner for ten to fifteen minutes. Wash the face with cold water afterwards and stay indoors for at least an hour.

Sage improves the appetite and helps in the digestion of food by stimulating the flow of bile and digestive juices. Its tannin content relieves diarrhoea and minor gastric upsets. In particular, sage aids the digestion of fats, so the cheese Sage Derby may be a good choice for those who find cheese slightly indigestible. I use the young leaves in salads with beans.

Tea for insomnia

Sage tea can be taken at bedtime for insomnia. Pour one pint of boiling water on to one ounce of the dried herb and take half a cupful as required. A more pleasant drink is made by mixing fresh sage (half an ounce of the leaves) with the juice of one lemon or lime, and a quarter ounce of grated rind, with honey or sugar to taste. Infuse in two pints of boiling water and strain after half an hour.

Sage also keeps the skin healthy and by toning and disinfecting the scalp it stops hair falling out. Chewing fresh sage leaves whitens the teeth. Try grinding sage and sea salt to make a tooth powder.

Sage for animals

A standard infusion of sage is excellent for coughs and chest infections in animals, even better than thyme. Powdered or mixed into small balls with honey it can be given as a pill twice a day to aid recovery and cleanse the system. It helps puppies with teething and, if they will stand it, will clean and freshen cats' and dogs' teeth.

Margaret Skinner

*B*irth and *A*fter

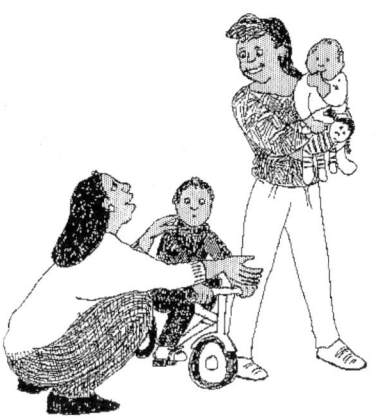

*'**M**atrozone Promotes
Natural, Rapid and Easy
Confinement. Ensures Healthy,
Beautiful, and Bright Children.'*

Advertisement c 1912

Pregnancy

Pregnancy is a strange condition. Perfectly innocuous food and drink suddenly become unpalatable or cause acute indigestion. Things don't get any better the second time around either.

Three months into my second pregnancy I knew I had to find a solution or die of a water and cream cracker overdose. My garden provided it. Melissa (lemon balm) and mint grow in abundance. A tisane made from fresh picked leaves after each meal was refreshing and did wonders for the heartburn. That was eight years ago, but I still drink it.

Geraldine Friend

....

A tea made of Red Raspberry Leaves, before and after confinement, is unequalled by any other agent. If the pains are premature it will make all quiet, and when they are timely it will occasion a safe and easy parturition. It is perfectly safe under all circumstances. If the mother is weak it will strengthen and cleanse her, and abundantly enrich the milk.

'Get Back to Nature and Live' C W Aloysius Browne
....

Egyptian beliefs

Doctors in ancient Egypt practised a method of determining in the early stages of pregnancy whether a woman would bear a boy or a girl. They put wheat and barley in a cloth bag and the woman urinated on them each day. If the wheat germinated, she would bear a boy; if the barley germinated she would bear a girl; if neither germinated the woman was not pregnant.

Women believed if they visited a birthing mother while wearing an indigo dress she would have no more children until she visited an indigo dye house.

Yorkshire customs

When I was a midwife in Yorkshire the mothers used to ask me to burn the placenta on the fire. Sometimes it would pop as it burned and they would count the number of pops because that's how many more children they would have.

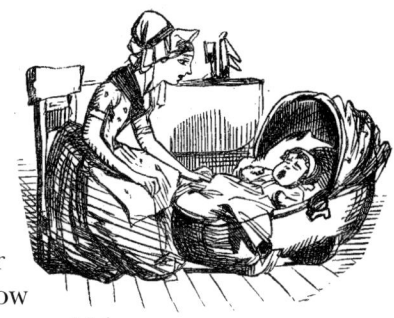

If a baby was born with a caul over its face, the midwife felt she had not delivered the baby properly. But cauls were considered lucky and sailors liked to have one since they were meant to prevent drowning. Only one baby I helped to deliver had a caul and the other nurse and I shared it. I have it still, it's like a piece of shrivelled-up plastic. But I haven't drowned.

Mollie Smith

Care for mothers and children

After the birth of my son, I was advised by my Italian mother to stay inside in the house for 10 days. It was winter and I was uncomfortable as I had stitches, so I did as she told me. This is probably a hangover from the days when women were in danger of becoming infected.

The Sri Lankan health visitor called round at a time when the baby had very bad congestion. She said that her mother told her to suck out the congestion and spit it out. Disgusting, but it does work.

The best way to treat nappy rash is simply by cleaning with cold water and drying well. My mother's Polish neighbour told me this and she herself was told it by a West Indian midwife in France!

The best advice I had was to trust my instinct.

Linda Maestranzi

Knowledge of life

The ladies of the Indian Yoga group in Reading practise Ayurvedic medicine. Dating back in India more than 5,000 years, Ayurveda means 'knowledge of life'. The principle is that disorder can be prevented as long as balance is maintained in the body, mind and spirit, so you must know yourself. The ladies talk about health in body and mind.

The mind and body are not separate. There are three modes of nature: sattva or activity, tamas or lethargy, and rajas or balance. Everyone is different – some might be more active, others more lethargic. The idea is to treat each person according to the mix, in order to achieve balance. In that state of perfect balance you should be able to experience the different types of joy: vata, pitta and kapha.

You give medicine according to the nature of the person. For example, a very active person would take garlic which brings down blood-pressure and is good for the heart. A lethargic person will find that onions liven the person up. A lively person will like hot, spicy things, food that is sour and salty, extreme tastes, alcohol. Food can cure so many things.

Germs are secondary. They will take root and flourish if the body is not healthy. If you have a very fatty diet – bacon, puddings and alcohol – germs will attack. Goat's milk and sheep's milk are healthier than cows' milk. They have smaller fat molecules.

Avoid salt particularly as you get older. Follow the body's instinct, ask yourself what you want to do.

Turmeric is one of the most powerful healing spices. If you have a sore throat in the summer, make a medicine of honey, a little hot ghee, some oregano and turmeric powder. It is both soothing and healing.

Put oregano, salt and turmeric, roast, ground and mixed in a bottle. A teaspoon is good for gastric trouble. A drink of turmeric, honey and water, preferably heated in a copper pot, is also good for the stomach.

One member of the group said: "My brother fell downstairs and had a big bump and my mother put turmeric powder and oil on the bump and it disappeared. I fell and broke the nail on my toe, it turned black and was very painful. I applied turmeric powder in oil, covered it in gauze and a bandage, then put a splint under my foot to support it and very quickly the swelling went down."

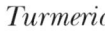

Turmeric

Another said she used turmeric and witch hazel on a sprained ankle, which cured it in two or three days, and another recalled how her grandmother used an ointment of pine resin, heated with turmeric, to ease a twisted ankle.

More advice: caraway seeds are good for you. You roast them slightly, pound them into a powder, mix with buttermilk and a pinch of salt and it stops diarrhoea. It clears the system and in 24 hours you are well again.

White pomegranate is also effective in cases of diarrhoea because you don't get dehydrated when you take it. There is something in pomegranate which gives strength, a feeling of vitality.

To treat dysentery, fry raisins in butter, and put them in milk with fenugreek seeds. When you are in India it is good to drink hot water and lemon with a bit of pepper first thing in the morning. That prevents dysentery or flu and keeps you healthy.

Ginger is a powerful spice. Scrape off the peel or rind, soak in water, grate it, and mix with some water, honey and lemon juice to make a drink which prevents flu.

More hints: Hot castor oil up the nose will help with a cold.

If you have smallpox, burn cow-dung, sieve the ashes, put them on the smallpox scabs and they disappear.

Use white lime on bumps and bruises, or eat it in betel leaves.

Drink two big cups of hot water before you sleep and when you wake up because it is good for the bowels.

For earache, warm oil and garlic and put a few drops in the ear.

Ginger

Some thoughts about childbirth:

After delivery, an Indian woman will lie on a bed of ropes under which is a fire of leaves and lamb- and calf-dung. The smoke rises and this helps back-ache.

Make little tampons from turmeric paste wrapped in muslin and dipped in oil. It prevents infection.

Take three types of bitter things, pepper powder, dry ginger powder and cinnamon, for eleven days after delivery and it gets the stomach back in shape.

Heat a stone in water and add dill and oregano to that water and give it as a drink to a new mother. It also helps bring the tummy down.

When you are feeding your baby, chew half a tea-spoon of oregano seeds three times a day and baby won't get wind. It is also good for asthma.

Massage the mother and baby twice a day with oil. A touch of saliva and mucus from the nose on the child's belly button will draw the gas out.

Swami Ambikananda, Kamala Tailor, Tarala Jagirdar,
Indira Desai, Panna Desai, Vijayalaxmi-Viji,
of the Indian Yoga Group, Reading

Child care in South Africa

There is a plant like wild rhubarb with hairy leaves in South Africa which was used by women who had had a baby. They would pound the roots, infuse them and use them as an enema or if there was trouble getting the placenta out. That would do it.

After birth, a woman who wanted to get her figure back in shape tied her stomach tightly to enable the muscles to knit together again. I think this sometimes pushed the stomach up awkwardly and created a hernia. However, if the woman had to grind the corn on the stone, her figure went back very quickly.

If a breast-feeding mother had a baby with thrush, especially little girls with vaginal thrush or oral thrush, they would spurt the breast milk on the infected place. They would so the same for conjunctivitis.

When the baby had a congested nose, the mother sucked the mucus out so it didn't settle on its chest. In America they have created little nasal aspirators to do the same thing.

Rose Cam

....

In Poland, in the old days, people would sometimes put a sick baby in the wood-burning oven while it was still warm (but not hot!) to help it sweat out its fever.

Ala Zolkiewka

....

Teething troubles

Senna and Rhubarb and Snails, with a mixture of prunes, to be used for Collick and Stomack aches, and to make the children's first teeth come out without paine.

The Boston Evening Post (1771)

Mothers in Pakistan

When you were ill in Pakistan, you didn't go straight
to the doctor. Most of the remedies were home-
made. Whenever a child was to be born, the grandmother would always come. There were servants to
do the work but she would be there to take special
care of the baby and the mother. It was her duty to
see that the mother was properly looked after for
40 days and during that time strangers were not
normally allowed in to see the little baby and the
mother in case they brought in
germs.

Special diets were pre-
pared for the mother to
give her strength. She
had extract of chicken
– the chicken was
boiled until even the
bones became soft.
Another dish was made of
semolina, fried in ghee, mixed
with almonds, sultanas, coconut and other dried
fruits, and she would have a few spoonsful with
every meal.

My grandfather was a hakim, treating patients with
herbs – people in those days would have their personal herbalist.

My grandmother had a special way of tending
new-born babies when they were going to bed. The
idea was that when the baby was in the mother's
womb it was in a closed space; after confinement it
finds itself suddenly in the wide world. My grandmother would get a strip of soft muslin and wrap
the baby in it before it went to sleep so that the
baby felt secure, as if it were still in the womb.

Babies were never left in a separate room to sleep.
They always slept in the same room as the mother,

in the same bed or in a cot, until they stopped breastfeeding or another child came along. The father had a separate room. The babies were never left alone but were with someone for 24 hours a day.

No matter how poor you were, you were brought up to think that having a baby was the best thing that could happen to a person. You were responsible for that child and you were not going to get married and have babies until you could look after them and support them.

Akhtar Aziz

Preserved by ashes

The ashes of the dung of a black cow, given to a new born infant, doth not only preserve from the Epilepsia, but also cures it. (c 1721)

'The Compleat English Dispensatory' Dr John Quincy

....

My brother and I had whooping cough and measles at the same time. We had a German doctor and he recommended we drank a glass of port each day. He came round and tested it!

Cyril Shuffle, 91

....

Mother knows best

I was very healthy and never caught anything as a child. When my brother caught chicken pox or measles my mother put me in the same bed so that I could catch it and get it over with – but I never did.

I remember I missed a prize because of that. We used to get a certificate at school for never being absent and in the last week of the year my brother caught measles so I was put in bed with him and missed school. I never got that certificate. My mother reckoned I must be a carrier because I never caught anything.

George Pottinger, 88

Passing on the disease

'... I went and made a visit to Mrs Graham, some-time Maid of Honour to the Queen-Dowager, now wife to James Graham, Esq., of the privy purse to the King; ... I returned to our inn, after she had showed me her house [Bagshot Park], which was very commodious and well-furnished, as she was an excellent house-wife, a prudent and virtuous lady....

'Her eldest son was now sick of the small-pox, but in a likely way of recovery, and other of her children run about, and among the infected, which she said she let them so on purpose that they might whilst young pass that fatal disease she fancied they were to undergo one time or other, and that this would be the best: the severity of this cruel distemper so lately in my family confirming much of what she affirmed.' (September 15, 1685)

John Evelyn (1620-1706), diarist

Women's health

Wise-woman

Digby Cole, the Reading herbalist, remembers an

old lady who used to live not far from Bockmer. Although she took care never to claim supernatural powers, she was regarded as a wise-woman and even in her extreme old age she was consulted on all imaginable topics. She used to warn people not to pick up a pin if they found it lying in the road, because a witch may have put it down when they saw someone coming. If anyone picked it up and kept it they would then be in the power of the witch.

She advised the young girls of Bockmer to wash their faces using distilled water of elder leaves which had been gathered in May.

The old lady kept in her cottage a supply of an ancient remedy which her mother had sold from door to door. A tattered label described this as: "The Golden Pills of Life and Beauty also known as the Trowbridge Pills. For the complaints incident to the female constitution. Prepared by Mrs. Jane Ludlow of Warminster."

'*Witchcraft in the Thames Valley*' Tony Barham

···

Mustard seed revives an hysterical woman.

Pliny, Roman historian (AD23-79)

···

Final word on exercise (Daily Mail, May 3, 1907)

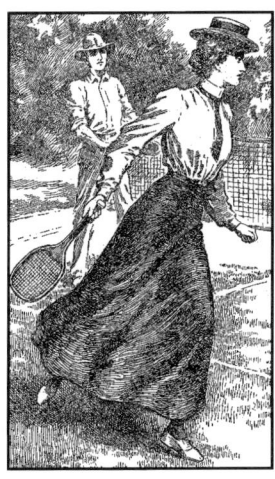

An old advertisement for Elliman's embrocation

Exercise is the only method – and I use the word only advisedly – open to a woman to obtain [the] lissomeness and delightful grace that is one of her truest charms...

Exercise that gives firmness to every part – the cheeks, the neck, the bust, the limbs – is a boon to beauty and a handmaid to youthfulness.

This exercise must however, be scientific exercise, and not the rough and tumble pastimes indulged in by the other sex. Games such as football, cricket, hockey are not – although I know many women will disagree with me – suitable for the gentler sex. Certainly if a woman wishes to keep young and fair to look upon she will not indulge in them. They may be healthy in a way – that is a moot point – but they have a distinctly coarsening effect upon both figure and complexion.

Herbal remedies in Poland

Like many European countries, Poland made great use of herbal remedies up to the beginning of this century. Many of the herbs were to be found in the woods and forests but these days they are protected species, and it is illegal to pick them. Here are some of the cures and treatments for a variety of common illnesses still used, I am sure, in country districts in Poland.

For ulcers, the juice of an onion, or the juice from the leaves of comfrey, *Symphytum officinale*, that most useful of plants, were taken. The comfrey leaves or those of thyme may also be put on gauze and used as a poultice for ulcers. For internal ulcers, such as stomach ulcers, the powdered root of comfrey, half a teaspoonful in water, four times a day, is very beneficial. My Polish herbal, Jan Muszynski's 'Medicine of the Countryside' (1956) does not say whether this will merely soothe the ulcer, or ultimately cure it.

Onion has a myriad of uses, both external and internal, not just as a flavour enhancer for food. Softened by a little gentle cooking (not frying), it is an excellent antibacterial medium, and may be used for dressing wounds and abscesses.

For those with a poor appetite, *Artemisia absinthium*, or wormwood, an infusion of the dried herb, was used. This was also used for gastro-intestinal pain and dyspepsia, but had to be carefully administered as too much or for too prolonged a time would be damaging. (Wormwood is a modern ingredient of vermouth.) Another herb with a similar use was *Menyanthes trifoliata*, or bogbean.

For colds, flowers of the lime tree, *Tilia europaea*, made into a tea, made a common and popular medicine. It was also used for headaches, and coughs and catarrh in children. An infusion of the bark was a popular remedy in France for lowering the temperature.

Raspberry leaves, and leaves of the willow, which contain salicin from which aspirin is derived, also helped to cool a fever. Willow bark or leaves steeped in wine and used as a wash was a cure for scurf and dandruff.

Matricaria chamomilla, or feverfew, helpedto soothe young children when teething. As its English name suggests, it was also beneficial for reducing fever. Mint and sage were used for teething troubles in infants, and juniper berries were believed to help liver disorders and arthritis.

Feverfew

Valerian is still used by a Polish lady of my acquaintance, Mrs Tola Boguszewicz, for her nerves, and she swears that using the plant as an infusion is far better than modern pills made from the plant. Unfortunately this plant is now very rare in the wild, both in Poland and Britain, and difficult to obtain.

Glycyrrhiza glabra or liquorice is made into a syrup with linseed oil from flax for dry coughs and hoarseness, especially for children. *Tussilago farfara*, or coltsfoot, is used as a syrup for asthma, as is thyme.

Finally, acne in teenagers can be cured by infusing half a teaspoonful of the powdered leaves of *Viola tricolor*, heart's-ease, or the wild pansy, in boiling water. This is drunk, rather than used as a wash.

Betty O'Rourke

*O*ut on a *L*imb

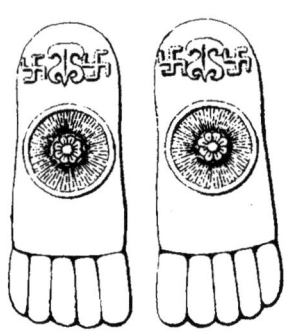

'*I*t has been computed that Bad
Legs have caused more
misery and suffering than all the
wars ever undertaken by the
world's rulers. – The Tremol
Treatment for Bad Legs.'

Advertisement c 1912

Limbs

Aches and pains

My grandmother would pick a type of lily and put the flowers in a jar with spirit. This was left for a while and then she used to rub it on to sore legs or to relieve the pain of rheumatism. Nettles are also good for this but you need a strong heart! Once when my father hurt his back he picked a big bunch and beat his back with them. It helped. He was able to go back to work but he said it was very painful and wouldn't do it again.

Joan Head, from Switzerland

....

For arthritic or muscle pain, rub nettle leaves on pain area. It stings but takes the pain away.

Trini Bello, from Spain

....

Soothing massage

People in Pakistan don't take tablets for aches and pains in their limbs. A woman would come nearly every day to give you a massage. This woman had no education but had learned her craft over the generations. She didn't charge but you would pay her with clothes or food.

Akhtar Aziz

Nettle

Virtues of celery

The virtues of celery in all cases of rheumatism are too well known to need repeating.

'Get Back to Nature and Live' C W Aloysius Browne

'Enter rheumatism'

'Enter rheumatism and takes me by the knee. So much for playing the peace-maker in a shower of rain. Nothing for it but patience, cataplasm [poultice or plaster] of camomile, and labour in my own room the whole day till dinner time – then company and reading in the evening.' (1827)

Sir Walter Scott (1771-1832)

'Right old verjuice'

'This day I visited Mr John Temple who gave me for my rheumatic pains a bottle of right old verjuice [the acid juice of green or unripe grapes, crab-apples or other sour fruit, expressed or formed into a liquor] and advised me to take a glass of it with a toast in it every morning fasting and going to bed and to rub my joints with it after it is well warmed, to continue this three weeks.'

The Earl of Egmont, 18th century diarist

Arms and hands

Cabbages and things

Quite recently a very dear friend called. She told me she had been diagnosed as having rheumatoid arthritis and was complaining of severe pain in the arm.

"Have you heard about the cabbage leaf cure?" I asked. "No," she said, "tell me". "You wrap the affected part in a cabbage leaf," I said.

She agreed to sit with her arm encased in a large leaf. As the leaf warmed with her body heat the smell was less than pleasant. After about an hour she announced there had been a reduction in pain.

Roisin O'Callaghan

For chapped hands (1907)

Take common starch and grind it with a knife until it is reduced to the finest powder. After washing the hands, wipe them and while they are still damp rub a little of the starch over them. The effect is most soothing. Mustard ground to a very fine powder and mixed with a little water is an excellent thing for cleansing the hands after handling strongly odorous substances such as onions and cod-liver oil.

....

When a child runs indoors crying because of his cold fingers, he usually rushes to the fire, holding his hands down to the heat. If the order is reversed and the hands held with the fingers pointing upwards for a few minutes, there will be no painful sensa-tions as the fingers grow warm. The reason is that when the fingers are held down the blood rushes into 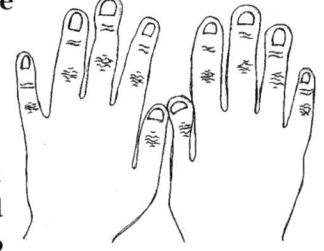 **them but when they are held upward, the circula-tion being more gradual, no pain is felt. (1907)**

....

Legs, knees and ankles

A drop of ouzo

Jan, on holiday in Rhodes, slipped while getting off a donkey in Lindos and sprained her ankle. The donkey owner immediately put the native drink, ouzo, on the ankle to bring out the bruise.

Daphne Barnes-Phillips

Snails in a bag

For poisoned elbow and knee, place snails in a bag with salad oil and paraffin. The liquid is applied to the joint affected.

Berkshire gypsy remedy

A case for Mr Browne

Herbalist W Aloysius Browne (1927) cures a case of synovitis of the knee (known as Housemaid's Knee)

"[One of my cases] was that of a dear little Sister of a Southampton Convent. The allopathic doctor had failed to cure her after three months' treatment. By the doctor's orders the Sister was kept in bed all the time and at the end of this period he announced to her that her only hope was to go to a Nursing Home and to have the knee in plaster and splints for five or six months.

"Now I think I ought to mention her parents had been paying for the doctor all this time, otherwise the Rev Mother would have certainly asked me to attend to this Sister.

"Now it happened that one afternoon I was at the convent attending to another Sister who was ill; and as the little Sister naturally did not fancy five or six months in the hospital, the Rev Mother asked me to see her, which I did.

"I told her I had never known in my 43 years' experience a failure. She then placed herself under my treatment. Looking out of the infirmary window into the grounds, I said to the Rev Mother: 'Look! there is any amount of Ragwort growing all around your grounds, and this herb is the finest for fomentation that one could possibly have.'

"So this was used, as well as the usual herbal remedies, and now they always gather the Ragwort and keep a supply for any cases requiring fomentation.

"This little Rev Sister was cured completely in less than four weeks; although I not only had to cure

the Synovitis but skin eruptions and abscesses created by the strong chemicals used on the knee by the
doctor's order.

"There is no doubt that the Synovitis was caused by
kneeling in prayer for so many hours on the knees,
on the hard wood. So I ordered her (by permission
of the Rev Mother) to keep her knee well in future
by always having a cushion to kneel upon."

First catch your pig

Ankle and wrist sprains should
be treated with grease from pigs,
specifically Large Whites.

*Mother Jame, a 19th century-
wise-woman*

Stopping leg cramps

Put corks in your bed.

Mollie Smith

....

**When the cramp is in the legs it is often an excel-
lent idea to place the limb against something cold,
such as the marble slab of the washing stand, and
always have hot water bottles in bed every night.**

'Get Back to Nature and Live' C W Aloysius Browne

....

Feet

Soldiers' drill

The snake apple tree which grows in southern
Africa has a small yellow fruit rather like a cherry
tomato. You can scrape off the skin and use the
juice on athlete's foot and fungal diseases. It was
used by soldiers in the bush during the Struggle
(the Zimbabwean war of independence) in the
1960s and 70s.

Jack Callow, Zimbabwe

Guzzunders

When I suffered from a chilblain on my little toe, my mother said that the best cure was to soak the foot in urine. Now, of course, today that would involve collecting the liquid but, in the 1950s, many people kept chamber pots under their beds to save themselves having to get up during the night and go downstairs to the toilet which was outside their house, even in large towns such as Reading where I was born and bred.

Imagine the disturbance of going downstairs, possibly by candle-light as we did not have electricity until I was about eight – before that my parents had to rummage for matches to light the gas-mantle. Add to that the cold – houses were heated during the day by coal fires and mostly only one in the main living room unless someone was ill – and the fact that, in one's sleepy state, it would be so easy to forget to lock up again after re-entering the house, you can quite understand why guzzunders were so popular.

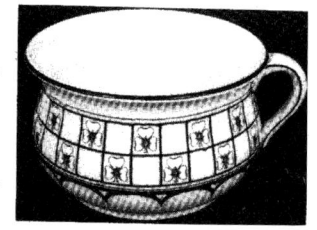

For those of you who have not come across this terminology, a guzzunder, following the usual euphemisms used for our bodily functions, is another name for a chamber pot as it "goes under" the bed!

Obviously, I wasn't too happy about trying this idea of soaking my foot in my own urine but it does seem to have done the trick as I do not recall suffering chilblains to this day!

Daphne Barnes-Phillips

The only cure for chilblains was putting your foot in the potty.

Cyril Shuffle, 91

An Infallible Remedy for Chilblains

Take one drachm of sugar of lead, and two of white vitriol, reduce them to a fine powder, and add four ounces of water. Before using this lotion, it is to be well shaken, then rubbed well on the parts affected, before a good fire, with the hand. The best time for application is in the evening. It scarcely ever fails the most inveterate chilblains by once or twice using. Not to be used on broken chilblains.

Fisher & Son's Money-getting Businesses (1849)

For chilblains, apply equal parts of turpentine and paraffin. (1907)

For a painful broken blister on a heel, my mother would carefully peel the thin membrane from inside an eggshell and cover the blister.

Audrey Cook

A New Zealander suffering from blistered heels while walking in the bush should find a flax plant and apply the jelly from the base of leaves, which are antiseptic, to the blister or place a leaf over the heel.

For corns

Peel the skin off a leaf of the little succulents called houseleeks and put it on the corn.

Mollie Smith

Bathe the Part, if not inconvenient, in Warm Water, and apply an ivy Leaf, previously steep'd for 24 Hours in Vinegar. Repeat the steep'd Leaf each Day, till the Corn is eradicated, and the Space it occupied becomes smooth, which in most cases will be a week.

From Mary Loder's recipe book (18th century)

The smell of Christmas

My grandmother knew a lot about herbs. She was the one who introduced them to me when I was growing up in St Kitts.

I like all herbs but at the moment my favourite is one called lemon verbena. It is pale green and a bit woody and comes from South America which is why it dies if you don't look after it. It has an absolutely glorious lemon-scented smell. You can use it dried for stuffing in things that will smell or as a tea for when you've got colds. Actually, I prefer smelling it to drinking it as a tea. Every time I pass it in the garden, or if I have one indoors, I squeeze the leaves to release the smell.

My next favourite is thyme. Aside from its aroma I use it to season food. You will find that herbs, like thyme, were used in hot countries to help to preserve the food before refrigeration.

The most common way in which I use herbs is in aromatherapy and oil of thyme is very strong. Its properties are antiseptic; it will help against viruses and it will promote the white blood cells which fight infection.

I always grow parsley, peppermint, sage, marjoram, chives, and garlic. I've still got some valerian – the slugs didn't seem to like them. With aromatherapy I use lavender a lot which is quite a common basic essential oil which I use every day.

The properties I like best about herbs are their aroma and the fact that they are

Peppermint – Mentha piperita

therapeutic, which means that they help to make people better. All modern medicines today are in some way synthesised from herbs so you will see that they have played an important part in their composition. Herbs were used centuries ago. The Persians liked the scent of roses and other sweet-smelling sources of oils for cosmetic uses. The Chinese, too, had their own various herbs.

How all this has come down to my grandmother, I don't know, but she knew a lot about herbs and put it to good use. Whenever we had colds she used to give us thyme teas.

She also gave us garlic tea. It tasted awful but nowadays we recognise how wonderful it is. It acts as a decongestant, getting rid of the mucus, and it helps to regulate the blood-pressure. It kills almost everything so if you have fungus problems – athlete's foot, and things like that – it will help.

Spearmint – Mentha viridis

We grew lemons and limes on the island where I was born, but not oranges, so at Christmas time we'd have to buy them and, as all people from poorer countries do, we'd use everything that we could.

We would peel all those oranges very carefully and put the peel out to dry. Then we'd use the rest of the fruit. You can make a very nice tea from oranges. When I came into aromatherapy, I found that there is an essential oil of orange. It smells wonderful and it is very cheering. The smell of oranges always makes me remember that pleasant Christmassy feeling.

Carol Shepherd answering questions from pupils at Reading Girls School

Desirable spice

Traditionally nutmeg was used to relieve rheumatic pain, as well as digestive and kidney problems, and it is believed to stimulate the circulation. Today it's more in demand throughout Europe and the Middle East as a culinary spice in both sweet and savoury dishes.

Nutmeg was known in Europe as early as Chaucer's time. It became seriously desirable after the Spice Islands (the Moluccas) were discovered in the 16th century and the great European trading nations feuded with each other to control imports. Its antiseptic properties made it one of the essential ingredients in medicinal remedies and for pomanders, which were used not only to disguise unpleasant smells but also to protect the wearer from lurking infections.

It's possible that the incredible medieval popularity of this seemingly innocuous tropical fruit was due more to the fact that it contains myristicin, a chemical with similar properties to certain psychedelic drugs. However, seekers of an out-of-body experience should be aware that raw nutmeg must be eaten in enormous quantities before any hallucinogenic or euphoric symptoms can be felt, and overindulgence could cause unpleasant side effects, including palpitations, nausea and convulsions. More pleasantly it is used in perfumes, and its evocative scent makes it a popular choice, along with other seasonal ingredients like cinnamon, frankincense and orange, for perfuming the home at Christmas.

Nutmeg

Linda Barlow

Appendix

'*To the sick – the suffering – to every man and woman victim of organic disease – local trouble or broken general health – Dr Kidd's offer of free treatments is given in the absolute faith and sincere belief that they can and will stop disease, cure it, and lift you up again to health and vigour.*'

American advertisement c 1909

Superstitions and beliefs

Dressed for health

New Englanders believed that if they wore nutmeg on a string or necklace it would prevent lice or boils, a corn-kernel necklace would prevent or cure headaches, and salt pork worn round the neck would ward off chills and colds.

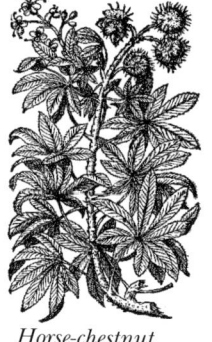

They believed a ring of dried raw potato peels worn on the middle finger of either hand would ease the pain of arthritis as would a horse-chestnut carried in the pocket.

Puritan boys and girls wore tansy bags around their necks and pressed to the chest all winter long to protect themselves from rheumatism.

Horse-chestnut

Adults ate the tansy root for gout.

··

In ancient Egypt beer, along with vegetable gum, was the principal remedy of Egyptian doctors. One Pharaoh left a message on his tomb which read "A delicious remedy against death is half an onion in beer foam."

··

Cure for cholera

During August 1849 an outbreak of Asiatic Cholera led to the death of 48 people [in a small hamlet called Gibraltar, near Dinton, in Buckinghamshire]. One of the few families who escaped the terrible epidemic attributed their safety to a long string of onions hanging up in the living room.

The onions showed signs of decay and the family were quite convinced that the cholera had attacked the onions, leaving the household unharmed.

'Witchcraft in the Thames Valley' Tony Barham

Willow Warding Spell

Willow is supposed to protect your family from harm and bring country freshness to the homes of town and city dwellers.

Take: an oil burner, 15 ml of almond oil, two drops each of rosemary, geranium and frankincense oils, three willow branches for cleansing, a potted red or white cyclamen plant, a new white candle.

On a night of a waxing moon, burn the oils in the burner and bear it through all the rooms of your house to cleanse them. Wave the willow branches through the smoke from the oils to spread their cleansing power.

Come to the room where the family most often gathers to perform the next part of the ritual. Place the oil burner and the

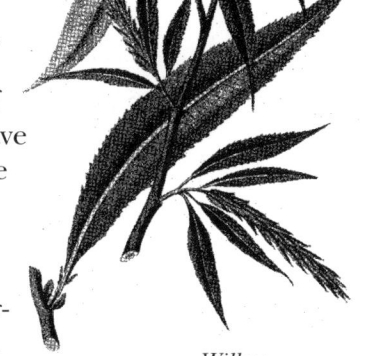

Willow

three branches on a table with the cyclamen and the candle. Light the candle. In your mind, take the light and spin it around the room like a tornado. Whirl it around each member of the family (including yourself) to cleanse away all negativity.

Taking no chances

One woman I looked after when I was a district nurse would never have her mattress turned on a Friday because it was bad luck. If it was Friday the 13th she wouldn't get out of bed.

Another lady I knew used to hibernate for the winter. She went to bed in October and stayed there cared for by her husband until April when she got up full of energy and spring-cleaned the house.

Mollie Smith

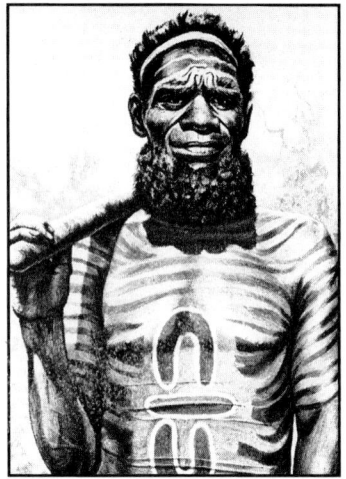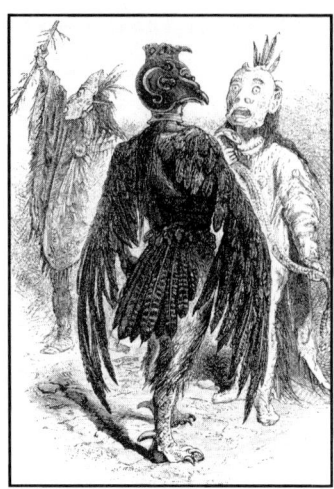

*Medicine men – (left) The wizard of Worgaia, a great medicine man
from central Australia; (right) three North American Indian medicine
men in ritual costumes.*

Wellcome Institute Library, London

Cure by steel and fire

Abdullah from Muscat, Oman, a student at the
University of Reading, has a large scar below his
ribcage and above his belly button, and several
smaller ones on his shoulders and back. These are
as a result of burns from red-hot knife blades and
screwdrivers applied to his skin when he was only
five years old. Several adults held him still while the
burn was made by a local Muscat healer.

The healers gain regional reputations for knowing
where to apply the red-hot tools to effect cures for
ailments. The practice is now dying out because of
modern western medical techniques and Abdullah's
younger brothers have fewer scars.

This used to be a widespread practice as the
Penny Magazine (May 1840) reports: 'External stim-
ulants have formed part of the practice of the physic
from the earliest times. One is the use of the red-
hot iron or cautery. Hippocrates says. "What medicine does not cure, steel cures; what steel does not

cure, fire cures; but what fire does not cure is incurable." The practice was common as irons were regularly heated for the round of the surgeons at St Bartholomew's Hospital.'

John Holden

Keeping healthy

Hints from W Aloysius Browne (c 1930)

Baths
Cold baths are splendid for those in good health, but should not be indulged in for long periods or by anybody in poor health.
Breath (offensive)
Take two charcoal tablets after each meal and nibble orris root. See to the stomach, teeth and liver.
Cloves
These will stop a craving for drink.
Exercise
Always avoid violent exercise, as this tends to bring about serious kidney troubles.
Infection
Remember infection first attacks the stomach. Keep the mouth closed as much as possible.

A turn -of-the-century advertisement for Elliman's embrocation

Sick room
To keep the air pure in a sick room wet a cloth in lime water and hang it in the room, and always note never to whisper near a sick patient.
Sugar
A most harmful food when taken to excess, especially for liver and kidneys. In diabetes if a patient takes sugar it means death, perhaps in a twelvemonth. Need more be said?

Advantages of Tobacco Smoking

Why should men smoke? There are some good reasons. Many break off from a brain-concentrating occupation for a smoke who would probably enjoy no interval at all otherwise...

Smoking helps the subject to rest. Sedentarily employed, a man may be induced to sit for many hours during the day without enjoying an interval, if he has nothing to break off for.

But a cigarette or pipe will give him occasion to put his hands in his pockets and walk up and down the room, or may induce him to go out of doors a little, so that he may obtain a pleasant and reinvigorating change from labour. Were he to merely stop his routine work and do absolutely nothing, his thoughts would be certain to wander back to duty again, and both he and his work would suffer in the end.

From 'The Secret of Good Health and Long Life'
quoted in the Daily Mail (February 17, 1899)

The Healthy Watchmaker

'Johnson the Watchmaker I called on this morning. I asked him how he preserved his health being so constantly employed in a sedentary business. He said by abstemiousness. That He never eats so much as He could, and when He finds himself a little indisposed He reduces the quantity of his usual allowance. He never takes Physick. He eats water gruel for breakfast – drinks half a pint at night.

He scarcely knows what it is now to feel very hungry. Sometimes He is low and faint with a sinking of the stomach: but rest from business for a day restores him.

He drinks a glass of cold water every morning when He gets up. Dr Fothergill of Bath told him that would carry off accumulating bile.' (1796)

Joseph Farington (1747-1821), landscape painter

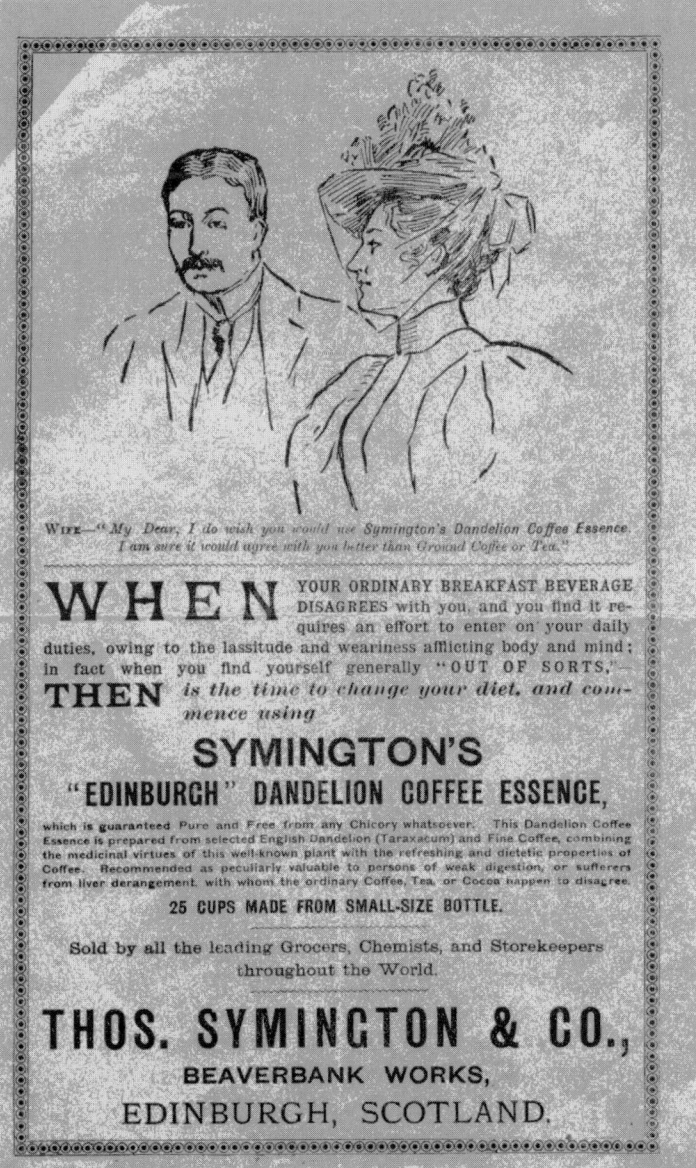

*An advertisement from the turn of the century for
Symington's Dandelion Coffee Essence.*
Fom the archives of GR Lane Health Products Limited

Every day and in every way

M. Emile Coué, the exponent of healing by auto-suggestion, interested the whole of Great Britain in 1922 with his curative formula, 'Every day and in every way I am getting better and better'. He claimed that the mere repetition of it would ultimately affect the body and bring it back to good health. His cure, he asserted, was the result of imagination, the most powerful influence about us. He was not a physician but a former apothecary, who in later years devoted himself to hypnotism and suggestion.

He attributed his general good health to the repetition of his own formula. (M Coué died in Nancy aged 69 in 1926.)

Daily Mail July 3, 1926

How fancy works

'I bless God I never have been in so good plight as to my health in so very cold weather as this is, nor indeed in any hot weather, these ten years, as I am at this day, and have been these four or five months. But I am at a great loss to know whether it be my hare's foot, or taking every morning of a pill of turpentine, or my having left off the wearing of a gown.' (December 31, 1664)

'Homeward, in my way buying a hare, and taking it home, which arose upon my discourse today with Mr Batten, in Westminster Hall, who showed me my mistake that my hare's foot hath not the joint to it; and assures me he never had his colic since he carried it about him; and it is a strange thing how fancy works, for I no sooner handled his foot, but I became very well, and so continue.' (January 20, 1665)

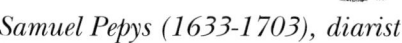

Samuel Pepys (1633-1703), diarist

Index

Printed in Great Britain
by Amazon